VAGINAL BIRTH AFTER CESAREAN

. . . .

The Smart Woman's Guide to VBAC

ELIZABETH KAUFMANN

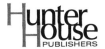

Hunter House
PUBLISHERS

Library of Congress Cataloging-in-Publication Data
Vaginal birth after cesarean : the smart woman's guide to VBAC /
Elizabeth Kaufmann.
p. cm.
Includes bibliographical references and index.
ISBN 0-89793-202-1 (pbk.)
1. Vaginal birth after cesarean. 2. Cesarean section—Popular works. I. Title.
RG761.K38 1996
618.4—dc20 96–16960
CIP

618.4
Kauf
PB

······························· ·····························..

Cover Design: Brenda Duke   Book design: *Qalagraphia*
Project Editor: Lisa E. Lee   Production Manager: Paul J. Frindt
Copyeditor: Mali Apple   Proofreader: Susan Burckhard
Marketing: Corrine M. Sahli   Promotion & Publicity: Kim A. Wallace
Customer Service: Joshua Tabisaura
Publisher: Kiran S. Rana

Printed and bound by Data Reproductions Corp., Rochester Hills MI
Manufactured in the United States of America

9 8 7 6 5 4 3 2 1   First edition

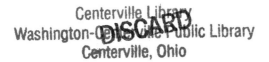
Vaginal Birth After Cesarean

This book is written for women and their health care providers about all the issues surrounding a birth after cesarean. In straightforward, unbiased terms, it explains:

- How a VBAC differs from a regular vaginal birth and how you can prepare for one

- What the medical risks and side effects are for repeat cesarean and VBAC, and how you can accurately assess them for yourself

- How to choose the right caregiver whether an obstetrician or a midwife and how to negotiate with them to get what you want

- How to overcome feelings of powerlessness and feel confident in the decisions you're making

- The history of cesareans: why the number has risen in the United States and around the world, and why there is now a movement to decrease cesareans and increase vaginal births

- What the current trends are among hospitals and insurers, and how they can affect you

Contents

· · · · · ·

Dedication

To my husband, Ernie Tucker, whose exceptional parenting and involvement with our children greatly facilitated this project, and whose emotional support bolstered me through the difficult moments. And to our two sons, Travis and Cameron, who unwittingly provided the genesis of this book, one of many great gifts they have given in the course of their young lives.

· · · · · ·

Important Note

The material in this book is intended to provide an overview of vaginal birth after cesarean section. Every effort has been made to provide accurate and dependable information. However, you should be aware that professionals in the field may have differing opinions and change is always taking place. Your health care and prenatal care should be undertaken with the guidance of a licensed health care practitioner. The author, editors, and publisher cannot be held responsible for any error, omission, professional disagreement, outdated material, or adverse outcome that derives from use of any of the procedures described herein.

......

Acknowledgments

My gratitude and utmost respect go to Phyllis D. Marx, M.D., who critiqued the manuscript, gave it medical credibility, and advised me of better ways to say things. Her gentle touch, receptive mind, and quick sense of humor make her an exceptional clinician who listens without arrogance, an excellent teacher, and a great role model for women in health care.

My deepest thanks to my friend and talented book editor, Carol Summerfield, who demystified the book-publishing world for me and who helped shaped the proposal, find the publisher, and review the contract, among other important things. She also believed in the worthiness of the project and in my ability to write it.

My thanks, too, to Lisa Lee, my editor at Hunter House, for embracing the project and supporting me the entire way. Her consistency, calmness, patience, and upbeat but informed approach make her a joy to work with.

My editors at *Shape* magazine and *Shape Fit Pregnancy*, Barb Harris, Peg Moline, and Michele Kort, helped considerably by publishing shortened versions of two chapters, for which I thank them.

I am very grateful to all the women who took the time to fill out surveys and share their fascinating birth stories. I'd like to name them, but promised anonymity—they will recognize themselves by their accounts. They very much fueled this project, and I appreciate the trust they placed in me.

I would like to thank the many people who directed me to the survey women and the friends who gave their support in other ways, including Jennifer Parmelee, Lee Green, Sally White, Sandra Fontánez-Phelan, Lisa Van Divender, Alison Davis, Magda Krance, Susy Schultz and the members of the Moveable Feast Book Group.

A number of medical doctors gave generously of their time and expertise, including Michael Socol, James Scott, Roneen Blank, Bruce Flamm, Maurice Abitbol, Alex Tulsky, Karyn Herndon, and Joanna Cain. I would also like to thank anthropologist Carol McClain, childbirth educator Nicette Jukelevics, and my excellent anatomy and physiology professor, Pat Duffie, at Loyola University in Chicago, for their help with various facets of the book.

I would like to thank the many people at the National Center for Health Statistics, the Centers for Disease Control and Prevention, the American College of Obstetricians and Gynecologists, and the American College of Nurse-Midwives for their patience and help in answering questions.

Last, but not least, thanks to my mom, Betty aka "Goggi" Kaufmann, my brothers C. B. and Rod Kaufmann and sisters-in-law Patty and Judy Kaufmann, and my mother-in-law, Peg aka "Mootie" McElroy, for their support and encouragement.

. . . . . .

Foreword

As the practice of medicine nears the end of the twentieth century, I find myself, as a physician, facing challenges that I never even dreamed of when I graduated medical school in 1980. At that time the first case of AIDS had yet to be reported, Managed Care Medicine was in its infancy, and everyone who underwent a cesarean section was destined for a repeat cesarean in their subsequent pregnancies. It was a time when patients expected their physicians to tell them what to do, not to give them choices. But medicine has changed, the attitudes and roles of both physicians and their patients have changed, and we all must make adjustments.

Throughout the evolution of this manuscript, Elizabeth Kaufmann has given me many opportunities to think about improving ways to approach prenatal patients who have experienced a previous cesarean section. The individual patient can easily become lost in the day-to-day workings of a busy obstetrician's office. However, each patient has her own needs, fears, desires, and medical and emotional issues to resolve. On one hand, the physician's innate competitive nature may drive her to strive for a lower cesarean section rate or a higher VBAC rate than her colleagues, but is that always the best thing for the individual patient? We, as obstetricians and midwives, cannot forget that we are in a unique partnership with our pregnant patients, and a significant percentage of our responsibility lies in educating these patients about their realistic choices. By doing so we hope that they can intelligently participate in their own decision-making processes.

In counseling women on whether or not to attempt a vaginal birth after a cesarean section, it may be difficult to clearly separate opinion from fact, the subjective from the objective, emotion from wisdom. This text uniquely presents the scientific data backing all the possible choices. Additionally, strategies for decision making are suggested, and women who have actually made these decisions share their experiences with the reader. If all of my previous cesarean patients were to read this book before coming to me to discuss their questions and concerns, perhaps patient anxiety would be significantly reduced due to their enhanced education. I expect that each of you who reads this book will be more secure in the decisions you make.

On behalf of women giving birth and their health care professionals, thank you, Liz!

Phyllis D. Marx, M.D.

Phyllis D. Marx, M.D., is an assistant professor of clinical obstetrics and gynecology at Northwestern University Medical School in Chicago. She is in private practice in obstetrics and gynecology in Evanston and Skokie, Illinois. She also works as a clinical investigator for the Chicago Center for Clinical Research.

Introduction

A friend who was pregnant with her first child recently asked me an innocent enough question.

"Why does it matter if someone has a vaginal delivery or a cesarean," she asked, "as long as the baby is okay?"

"You mean, why does it matter to someone other than the woman?" I responded.

"Yes."

"Because there's a national drive to lower the cesarean rate."

"Why?" she asked. A very good question.

"It's complicated," I said, "but cesareans are typically more expensive than vaginal births, so much of the reason behind it is economics. That's also why women are being kicked out of the hospital so quickly now after delivering. If cesareans were cheaper, I doubt that would be an issue."

"Oh," she frowned. "Using pregnant women to save money. That figures."

Most women go into their first pregnancy hoping and preparing for a vaginal birth. Anyone who has attended Lamaze classes knows that. When someone ends up with a cesarean, she may feel terribly disappointed at one end of the spectrum, incredibly relieved at the other. A woman's feelings afterward are complex, and she comes away knowing much more about childbirth than she did before. She may view labor and delivery differently. It is no longer safe to assume that every woman who has had a cesarean wants and hopes for a vaginal birth in her next pregnancy.

Today, most women who have had a cesarean can choose to attempt a vaginal birth after cesarean (VBAC) in their next pregnancy. This is a wonderful new option, and it signals the end of the 80-year-old dictum "Once a cesarean, always a cesarean."

VBAC is a great alternative if it is what you want. But the fact that it exists does not mean all women want it or even that it is right for all women. This aspect of the drive to lower the cesarean rate disturbs me: as the pendulum swings the other way, a new edict is taking hold, which could be called "Once a cesarean, now a VBAC." Rather than being viewed as an option, attempting VBAC is gradually becoming an expectation. Once again, women are being told what to do.

If there were only one viable medical option, a clearly superior choice, such a directive might make sense. However, elective repeat cesarean is also a fine alternative and a more time-tested one. And, in fact, studies show that 50 percent of women who are offered a VBAC prefer repeat cesarean. Being pressured to have a VBAC does not sit well with such women, just as being pressured to have an elective repeat cesarean does not sit well with women who prefer to try VBAC.

Unfortunately, a doctor is trained to try to shape and control your decision and not necessarily to thoroughly inform you of the choices, listen to your concerns, and work out an acceptable agreement with you. What most women need from a doctor is a partnership, and you can get it if you try.

The aim of this book is to inform you of the pros and cons of both VBAC and repeat cesarean and to help you formulate a decision with which you feel comfortable. Unless you regularly read obstetrical journals, most of this material will be new to you. This book will also help you get the most out of your relationship with your obstetrician or midwife. And unless you have talked to lots of mothers who have had a VBAC, and mothers who have tried, only to end up with a repeat cesarean, you may not have a sense of what it is like. In Part Two of this book, you will hear directly from women in different parts of the country who have had a VBAC, as well as from women who labored and ended up with another cesarean. You will also hear from women who had an elective repeat cesarean. If you already know what you want, this book will help you to get it.

The birth process rarely proceeds exactly as you imagine it will. But there are many choices along the way that you can exercise, if you know what they are. This book will help you maximize that power of choice.

PART ONE

. . . .

The Medical Scene

ONE

· · · ·

The Drive to Lower
the Cesarean Rate

Expectant mothers with an ear to the ground have heard the warning mantra: "Your chances of ending up with a cesarean are one in four. Don't be caught unaware. Do what you can now to avoid unnecessary surgery."

Mothers who have already had a cesarean and are pregnant again have undoubtedly heard about the VBAC option—that is, vaginal birth after cesarean. They may feel delighted or even vindicated to have this alternative. Or they may feel confused, pressured, or undecided. Some may feel guilty for preferring to have another cesarean, especially in light of all the negative publicity about the high cesarean rate.

It is VBAC candidates, in particular, for whom this book is written. At the same time these women may be feeling uncertain about which option to choose, others with strong opinions will be trying to influence their decision (even more than is the norm in pregnancy). Many medical studies have been conducted about VBAC, but few have looked seriously at the point of view of the women doing the birthing. Not many, if any, objective books have been written on the topic specifically for women. Many reports singing the praises of VBAC assume that you *should* try a VBAC and you *will* try a VBAC, regardless of how you feel about it. Contrary to that position, this book is pro-choice. A mother who has had a prior cesarean should be able to choose whether she wants to try a VBAC or to have a repeat cesarean. Do not assume that everyone you encounter takes this choice for granted.

How Did the Cesarean Rate Get So High?

Out of the blue, it would seem, the cesarean rate rose from just 5.5 percent of all births in 1970 to a high of 24.7 percent in 1988. That year, about 966,000 of 3,910,000 babies born in the United States were delivered by cesarean (see Table 1). Some are calling it a "cesarean epidemic." Doctors, insurers, national policymakers, consumer watchdogs, and cesarean-prevention groups all agree: the cesarean rate in this country is too high, still, even though it has plateaued.

Accompanying this sentiment is often a sense of moral outrage, replete with accusations that women are being ripped off, denied the true and natural experience of childbirth. Some would say it's no different from all those unjustified hysterectomies to which our mothers were subjected!

The loudest protest of all, however, is coming from the contingent who think that too many health care dollars are wasted delivering babies by cesarean. "It is unconscionable that every day unnecessary cesarean surgery is performed on thousands of women, squandering valuable millions of health care dollars, while almost 40 million Americans lack basic health insurance," write Mary Gabay and Sidney Wolfe, M.D., in *Unnecessary Cesarean Sections: Curing a National Epidemic,* published by Public Citizen's Health Research Group (1994). The group estimates that nearly half of all the cesareans performed in 1991 were unnecessary and that these excesses cost our society more than $1.3 billion.

Let's step back and take an objective look at how the cesarean rate got so high. Doctors have been accused of performing excessive operations because they have traditionally earned more for a cesarean than a vaginal birth. Also, a cesarean is sometimes more convenient for the doctor because it saves the time of waiting for the woman's labor to progress. But it would be too simplistic and too cynical to attribute the entire increase in the cesarean rate to the greed and convenience of doctors. In any event, some insurance companies have started to equalize physician reimbursements for vaginal and cesarean births to remove the profit incentive.

Table 1 The Cesarean Rate				
Year	Live Births	Cesareans Number	Percent	Repeat Cesareans Number	Percent

Year	Live Births	Number	Percent	Number	Percent
1993	4,039,000	921,000	22.8	336,000	36.5
1992	4,084,000	964,000	23.6	359,000	37.2
1991	4,111,000	966,000	23.5	338,000	35.0
1990	4,158,000	977,000	23.5	351,000	35.9
1989	4,041,000	962,000	23.8	342,000	35.6
1988	3,910,000	966,000	24.7	351,000	36.3
1987	3,809,000	929,000	24.4	328,000	35.3
1986	3,757,000	905,000	24.1	310,000	34.3
1985	3,761,000	854,000	22.7	295,000	34.6
1980	3,612,000	596,000	16.5	178,000	29.9
1975	3,144,000	327,000	10.4	89,000	27.1
1970	3,731,000	205,000	5.5	52,000	25.2

Source: Centers for Disease Control and Prevention. Morbidity and Mortality Weekly Report; April 21, 1995; 44(15) based on National Hospital Discharge Survey data.

Many doctors in turn blame the fear of lawsuits for the skyrocketing cesarean rate. It is no secret that we live in the most litigious society in the world. The fear of a malpractice claim certainly has contributed to the rising cesarean rate. Considering that some 80 percent of the malpractice suits filed against obstetricians involve failure to perform a cesarean, it's easier to understand why doctors have resorted to them more frequently. Doctors believe that cesareans can and do save the lives of babies and mothers, a fact that often seems overlooked in the cesarean debate today. However, the fear of malpractice litigation doesn't explain why the cesarean rate has also risen astronomically in countries such as Brazil and India, where such lawsuits are much rarer.

There are a multitude of other reasons for the increase in cesarean deliveries. Consider some of the relatively recent technological advances in obstetrics, including the popularization of electronic fetal monitoring; the gradual replacement of general anesthesia in cesarean birth to epidural or spinal anesthesia, which allows for greater participation of both parents in the birth experience; major improvements in prenatal care; the ability to diagnose fetal congenital problems in utero and sometimes intervene before birth; and remarkable improvements in neonatal intensive care that have allowed otherwise doomed babies to survive.

All of these developments came on the scene in the past thirty years, during the time the cesarean rate escalated. Some contributed directly to the cesarean rate. All have helped to improve childbirth outcomes, especially for babies.

"Beginning in 1969 and continuing through 1983, there was a sharp decline in fetal mortality," writes Diana B. Pettiti, M.D. "It has been claimed that many factors including increased use of family planning, increased availability of abortion, Medicaid, neonatal intensive care units, electronic fetal monitoring, and the rising cesarean section rate have caused the decline in fetal mortality starting in 1969, but it has not been possible to establish the contribution of each factor to the decline."

Outcomes have improved to the point that most of us expect to have perfect babies and speedy recoveries from birth. Yet complaints abound from women, and even some doctors, about the high-tech, low-touch, high-intervention mode of birth that now predominates in America. Machines have supplanted human hands. Where soothing voices once reassured the anxious mother throughout labor, now there's a void, or a continuous lumbar epidural. Unfamiliar attendants flit in and out of the room, poking and prodding as they see fit. A woman is lucky to get the doctor she wants and knows best from pregnancy, and doubly lucky if the doctor shows up before labor reaches a crescendo. Expectant fathers or friends trying their best to offer support are often lost in the labor-and-delivery-room maze, childbirth classes notwithstanding, especially during the first birth.

Not surprisingly, a counterrevolution to the high-tech mode of birth has also surged, as evidenced by the new fascination with midwifery, which is attracting an increasing percentage of expectant mothers with each passing year. Midwives and their patients embrace the human and natural elements of birth. Childbirth is not an illness or a medical condition to them but a positive, uplifting event that works quite well more often than not if left to its own devices. Midwives try to keep the interventions at bay. Not surprisingly, midwives have a lower cesarean rate than doctors, though they tend to care for women who are low risk.

Ultimately, women must choose between the typical hospital scenario with an obstetrician, where they will be expected to tolerate the interventions and forgo some of the human element, and the midwife experience, where they may not have as much technical support (especially if a physician isn't close at hand) but will have more human affirmation (see Chapter 6). This is a difficult decision for anyone who is expecting, and even more difficult for someone contemplating VBAC, who is by definition at higher risk for complications. Most midwives gladly take on women who want to attempt VBAC.

Some people argue that industrialized countries, such as Ireland, have experienced a decline in fetal mortality without as dramatic an increase in the cesarean rate as the United States has seen, and that therefore some of our increase must be unnecessary. These critics say cesareans can't be credited with dramatically improved outcomes. Maybe they are half right. At the National Maternity Hospital in Dublin, an active-management-of-labor program succeeded in keeping cesarean rates close to 5 percent in the eighties. But that program also incorporated a nurturing component that is woefully lacking in most of our management programs: continuous one-to-one care provided by a nurse midwife.

The important point here is that the birthing trade in the United States is deeply entrenched in technology, and most of us take the benefits of this technology for granted. To say it is time to drastically cut back the cesarean rate without closely reexamining all the concomitant advances is shortsighted in the absence of a reexamination of the other trends that are so closely intertwined. It's a little like saying we should turn off our fax machines, curtail overnight mail deliveries, and go back to relying on the U.S. postal service.

Women who schedule elective cesareans are blamed for copping out, for choosing convenience—yet what are all the sleek devices in the delivery room for if not for the convenience of doctors and hospitals? Not much remains of the "natural" in hospital childbirth, birthing rooms notwithstanding.

What we need to be asking is, if we still believe in the high-tech path that led to the 25 percent cesarean rate, why are we now saying that the cesarean rate is too high? Is it primarily because cesareans cost more than vaginal births? Is that a good reason?

Does it make sense to designate a particular number as the correct and desirable cesarean rate? Whose job is it to say this cesarean was reasonable, that one was not? If the cesarean rate declines, will outcomes get worse, get better, or stay the same? If we agree to lower the cesarean rate, how do we make sure it doesn't compromise the safety of mothers and babies?

Medical Developments and the Cesarean Rate

At least two medical advances, electronic fetal monitors and epidural anesthesia, have been blamed for contributing significantly to the rising cesarean rate.

Electronic fetal monitors track the baby's heart rate and print a continuous record of the rises and falls during contractions and the entire course of labor. Since 1970, electronic fetal monitors have almost universally replaced the older method of evaluating the baby's heart function, *intermittent auscultation*. That technique, preferred by some midwives today, involves placing a fetal stethoscope on the mother's abdomen and listening to the baby's heart rate.

The fetal monitor provides more information over the continuum of labor than intermittent auscultation, and a machine rather than a person takes the reading. But neither method is failproof, and fetal heart function is complicated. Heart rate can vary greatly in labor when everything is fine; it can also develop abnormalities that are fairly common during labor without compromising the baby. But prolonged drops in the heart rate or drops that don't

come back up after a contraction can also signal a serious problem, such as a deficiency in the baby's oxygen supply and the
inability of the baby to tolerate labor. Even for the most skilled
physicians, it can be difficult to tell for certain from the monitor,
or from intermittent auscultation, when something is wrong.

The faulty or overly cautious interpretation of the monitor
tracing has been blamed for excessive diagnoses of fetal distress
and, by extension, an excessive number of cesareans performed
due to fetal distress. In 1980, for example, when monitors were
used in less than half of U.S. births, the incidence of reported
fetal distress was just 1.2 percent of all deliveries. By 1992, when
monitors were used in three fourths of U.S. births, fetal distress
was reported in 9.4 percent of all deliveries. That year, fetal distress accounted for 10.5 percent of the cesarean rate. (Note that
there is often more than one reason for a cesarean. A woman who
experiences arrest of labor, for example, may also have a baby
with symptoms of fetal distress.) The question becomes, then, do
fetal monitors have a legitimate place in obstetrics?

"It's been known for awhile that the incidence of cerebral palsy
is about 2 in 1000 and the incidence of mental retardation about
4 per 1000," says Michael Socol, M.D., professor and head of
maternal-fetal medicine at Northwestern University Medical
School. "When electronic fetal heart rate monitoring came about
in the late sixties and early seventies, it was very logical to hope
that a more accurate assessment of fetal heart rate in labor would
allow obstetricians to intervene in a more timely way and decrease adverse outcomes. And to some extent it did in that there
was a decrease in intrapartum [during labor] stillbirths. So I think
electronic monitoring helped decrease the number of stillbirths in
labor. But what electronic fetal monitoring has not done is decrease the incidence of cerebral palsy or mental retardation."

Another potential drawback, Dr. Socol says, is that a monitor
requires the woman to remain on her back or side, positions that
may not favor vaginal delivery as much as if she were up and walking. Portable monitors that allow women to walk around are in
use in larger hospitals, though not typically in rural ones.

Despite these criticisms of monitors, however, few practitioners are seriously talking about abandoning them. We don't have anything better, yet. The existing alternative, intermittent auscultation, is supposed to be used only when the attendant-to-patient ratio is one to one, which can rarely be guaranteed in a labor and delivery ward. Most doctors still believe that the benefits of electronic fetal monitors warrant their use. If you are a VBAC candidate, unless you have a midwife, you can safely assume that you will be hooked up to a monitor. Monitors are believed to be the best device for providing a fast determination of a ruptured uterus. Although the incidence of rupture is low in the uterus scarred from a previous low transverse (horizontal) incision, this is the most worrisome risk to the VBAC mother (see Chapter 4).

Monitors are probably here to stay, but other measures can be taken to double-check whether a suspicion of fetal distress is founded. These are added interventions, of course. The less invasive but less reliable method is fetal scalp stimulation, which involves tickling or otherwise stimulating the baby's head. If the baby's heart rate increases in response, that is a reassuring sign.

The other technique is fetal scalp sampling, which involves pricking the baby's head for a blood sample and testing its acid-base status (pH). This gives a very accurate assessment of the baby's respiratory and metabolic condition and can be done in less than a minute. If the pH is reassuring, the baby is not suffering from fetal distress. Many doctors believe that fetal scalp sampling should be more widely used and that it could help to reduce the number of cesareans.

Another medical development that has been blamed for increasing the cesarean rate is epidural anesthesia. In particular, epidurals have been implicated for excessive claims of dystocia, or abnormal progress of labor, especially in first pregnancies.

One study found that women who received epidurals in their first labor had a higher incidence of both cesarean and forceps or vacuum-assisted deliveries than women who did not receive epidurals. Several features linked to epidurals were identified as potential contributors, including a decrease in uterine activity, a lengthening of the first or second stages of labor, and a decrease in the mother's urge or ability to push.

Obstetricians are well aware of these considerations, and there is an established tendency to expect extra time for women with an epidural to progress in their first labor. However, it is hard to argue a strong case against the most effective pain relief ever invented for labor, and epidurals are decidedly here to stay. Moreover, the content of the medication given in an epidural has evolved so that there can be less motor block—some motor control is needed for pushing—and yet equally effective pain relief.

Women who wish to avoid epidurals for fear of being too numbed or ending up with a cesarean don't have to have them, and women who choose a midwife aren't nearly as likely to get an epidural as those who choose an obstetrician. In fact, some midwives refuse to let their patients have one. However, many VBAC candidates who had an epidural in their previous labor would not consider attempting a trial of labor without the option of having one again. The American College of Obstetricians and Gynecologists, the leading association for ob-gyns, recommends that patients should be advised of the availability of epidurals because they may encourage more women to choose a trial of labor.

Other Reasons for the Rising Cesarean Rate

Breech deliveries

Breech presentation, or a different fetal position other than head down, occurs in 3 to 4 percent of all pregnancies. In 1980, only 67 percent of breech babies were delivered by cesarean. By 1993, 87 percent were delivered this way. Attempted vaginal delivery of a breech baby carries significantly greater risks to the baby as well as some additional risks to the mother. These risks haven't changed over time, but cesarean birth has become safer. Because cesarean birth is widely considered safer for breech babies, it is the norm today. Breech births and other malpresentations now account for 12.5 percent of all cesareans performed.

Forceps deliveries

The use of forceps to achieve a vaginal delivery has also declined, accompanied by an increase in the cesarean rate. According to a paper cited in *Williams Obstetrics*, a leading obstetrics textbook, forceps deliveries (also called *operative vaginal deliveries*) declined from 37 to 18 percent between 1972 and 1980, while the cesarean rate rose from 7 to 17 percent. The rate of forceps deliveries furthered declined to 4.3 percent in 1992, according to the National Center for Health Statistics.

Opinions about forceps and the frequency of their use vary widely from medical school to medical school and hospital to hospital. When used properly in the right circumstances, forceps can facilitate a vaginal delivery. Their inappropriate use can damage both mother and baby. Many medical schools no longer train residents in forceps use, a change some seasoned obstetricians lament. The fewer physicians that are trained in this technique, the more rapid the decline in expertise in its use. This, in turn, lowers the availability of forceps delivery as an alternative to cesarean.

One school of thought contributing to the decline of forceps use has held that a baby that does not come out spontaneously should be delivered by cesarean and that surgery poses fewer risks than forceps. This philosophy has certainly contributed to the rising cesarean rate. An alternative school holds that forceps and vacuum extractors can play an important role in a safe vaginal delivery if certain strict prerequisites are met—including that the baby's head has reached +2 station (see illustration page 42) and the cervix has dilated fully. When prompt delivery is called for, forceps may be used to rotate or pull gently on the baby's head to facilitate delivery. The vacuum extractor is preferred by some obstetricians today because it may cause less damage to the mother; reports show that effects on the baby are comparable.

It is difficult to predict the future of forceps and vacuum extractors and whether operative vaginal deliveries will make a comeback as the VBAC rate rises. However, it is clear that there is a relationship between the decline of forceps use and the increase of the cesarean rate.

Smaller families

People are having fewer children. This fact has changed the makeup of the population of pregnant woman. At any given moment, about half of the pregnant women in the United States are expecting their first child. Conditions that predispose a woman to having a cesarean are more common in women expecting their first child than in women who have had a previous vaginal delivery.

Older mothers

The number of women in their thirties and forties who are having babies has risen dramatically. According to the National Center for Health Statistics, the percentage of first babies born to women ages 30 to 39 increased fivefold in twenty years, from 3.8 percent in 1971 to 18.1 percent in 1991.

Maternal age is an independent risk factor for cesarean section. In 1993 in the United States, women ages 30 to 39 having their first baby had a 33.6 percent cesarean rate, and those from 40 to 49 had a 46.2 percent cesarean rate. By comparison, primary cesarean rates were 23 percent for women ages 25 to 29 and 20 percent for women ages 20 to 24.

Larger babies

Although low infant birthweight is still a problem in the United States, especially among black infants, it is also true that the birth of a baby weighing 9 or even 10 pounds is not as uncommon as it once was. Forty years ago, an 8-pound baby was considered large. Today, some doctors consider a weight of 4000 grams (8 lbs. 13 oz.) to be large, while others think a weight of 4500 grams (9 lbs. 15 oz.) or more to be large. In fact, the number of babies weighing more than 4000 grams increased from 8.4 percent in 1970 to 10.9 percent in 1990. The incidence of fetal macrosomia, or being large-bodied, appears to be on the rise, according to *Williams Obstetrics*. Moreover, the incidence of shoulder dystocia, or abnormal progress of labor due to difficult delivery of the shoulders, has increased in the past 20 years. The authors write that the likely cause is increasing birthweight.

The rise in birthweight is thought to be due to improved prenatal care and better nutrition during pregnancy. Several studies, including a recent one of more than 225,000 women in Washington State, published by Kiyoko M. Parrish, Ph.D., in the *Journal of the American Medical Association,* have concluded that increasing birthweight has contributed to higher cesarean rates. Other reports, however, say changes in birthweight have had minimal effect on the cesarean rate.

Repeat cesareans: The biggest culprits

Just a century ago, women rarely survived cesareans. They died of shock or bled to death because the medical community believed that stitching the uterus posed too great a risk of infection. The mortality rate declined somewhat after uterine sutures were introduced, but the rate of death from infection remained high until safer surgical techniques were pioneered in the early 1990s.

Still, cesareans were performed rarely, in the most dire of circumstances. In 1916, when Dr. Edwin Craigin of Columbia University made his famous statement "once a cesarean, always a cesarean," the cesarean rate was less than 1 percent. His statement was actually meant as an advisory not to perform a cesarean with a first baby unless it was absolutely necessary, because the mother would have to endure the risks of subsequent cesareans for any future pregnancy. At that time, cesareans were done with the classical, vertical uterine incision. This incision has a 12 percent chance of rupturing in a subsequent attempt to deliver vaginally, and such ruptures can be catastrophic to both mother and baby. Until the uterine incision was modified, Craigin's dictum about repeat cesareans was strictly enforced, and with good reason.

Over time, cesareans became very safe, and the mortality rate from cesareans is now negligible. By the mid 1970s, the classical vertical incision gave way to the low transverse (horizontal) uterine incision, which is used today in 90 percent or more of all cesareans. The scar from this incision has less than a 1 percent risk of rupturing in a subsequent labor because it is in a noncontracting part of the uterus. In time, this was considered a small enough risk to make VBAC a safe alternative.

Though Craigin's edict no longer applied, the majority of doctors still performed repeat cesareans as a rule. In 1983, the VBAC rate was a modest 4.6 percent.

The cesarean rate continued to rise in the 1980s, peaking at 24.7 percent in 1988. By that time, repeat cesareans numbered about 351,000 per year and accounted for more than one third of all cesareans. This sizable chunk became the single biggest target of the national crusade to lower the cesarean rate.

VBAC to the Rescue

In 1988, the American College of Obstetricians and Gynecologists issued strong new guidelines stating that women who had previously delivered by cesarean with a low transverse incision could safely attempt a vaginal birth in subsequent pregnancies. By that time, the research community had conducted numerous studies showing that VBAC was a safe alternative to repeat cesarean. The VBAC rate continued to increase, from 18.5 percent in 1989, to 20.4 percent in 1990, to 25.4 percent in 1993. This means that one out of four women with a prior cesarean are having a vaginal birth with their next baby.

Some people say these numbers represent progress. Change comes slowly in medical circles, especially when patients are exposed for the first time to unfamiliar or potential risks. It took ten years after low transverse incisions became the norm before the VBAC rate reached an even paltry 4.6 percent. The fact that it's greater than 25 percent ten years later is a good indication that VBAC is catching on.

Others say the VBAC rate has not risen fast enough. As part of a national health objective, the U.S. Department of Health and Human Services has called for a VBAC rate of 35 percent by the year

Table 2 The VBAC Rate		
Year	*Number VBACs*	*Percent VBACs*
1993	115,000	25.4
1992	119,000	25.1
1991	108,000	24.2
1990	90,000	20.4
1989	78,000	18.5
1988	50,000	12.6
1987	36,000	9.8
1986	29,000	9.5
1985	21,000	6.0
1980	6,000*	3.4*
1975	2,000*	2.0*
1970	1,000*	2.2*

*Based on too few deliveries to be statistically reliable.

Source: Centers for Disease Control and Prevention. *Morbidity and Mortality Weekly Report;* April 21, 1995; 44(15), based on National Hospital Discharge Survey data.

2000, along with a reduction in the overall cesarean rate to 15 percent. A recent federal vital statistics report says the VBAC goal may not be achieved, because the rate stabilized between 1991 and 1993.

Just as fingers have been pointed at various players for contributing to the rising cesarean rate, now there is an effort to find those to blame for the fact that the VBAC rate isn't higher. For one thing, some doctors have been slower than others to embrace VBAC or even to give their patients the option. Second—and this will come as a surprise to many—studies show that 40 to 50 percent of the women who are eligible for VBACs turn them down. Someone who has not undergone a lifesaving cesarean after a long labor might not understand this point of view. (This phenomenon is further explored in Chapters 3 and 5.)

Because of the national outcry over the high cesarean rate, however, women who are medically eligible for VBAC may find themselves under increasing pressure to attempt it. Some medical proponents of VBAC, including researchers and clinicians who have shown that VBAC is successful in 60 to 80 percent of the women who attempt it, now refuse to let patients elect a repeat cesarean. One Denver doctor I interviewed is extremely proud of his 83 percent VBAC rate, which is made possible in part by the fact that he refuses to care for patients who prefer an elective repeat cesarean, instead sending them to another practice.

"Although some women are being talked into unnecessary cesareans, many other women are demanding them," writes Bruce Flamm, M.D., a leading VBAC proponent and Riverside, California obstetrician who is research chairman for the health maintenance organization Kaiser Permanente. In other words, you may find yourself in a situation in which what you want is strongly challenged by your medical practitioner.

What would any medical battle be without the intrusion of everybody's favorite whipping boy—the health insurance company, particularly the health maintenance organization? As HMOs become increasingly involved with decisions that were once left to physicians, one thing they are doing in their relentless effort to contain costs is to mandate certain procedures and refuse coverage for others. Just as insurers instituted the recent drive to kick new mothers and babies out of the hospital in 6 to 12 hours—a move that prompted legislation in some states to limit that power—insurers are increasingly meddling in decisions regarding childbirth techniques and options. Some HMOs now refuse coverage for an elective repeat cesarean, insisting on a trial of labor in a subsequent pregnancy. It is important to know exactly what your coverage includes, ideally before you become pregnant.

If you become pregnant after having a cesarean, it may be taken for granted that you will want to attempt a VBAC. VBAC is a loaded topic, and everyone you encounter during your prenatal care will have an agenda for you, including doctors, midwives, hospitals, and insurance companies. What you ultimately need to remember is that it is your pregnancy and your child, and you don't have to let anybody take important choices away from you.

Medical Reasons for Cesarean Delivery

Regarding the innumerable and often overlapping reasons given for performing cesareans, an obstetrician recently wrote me, half tongue-in-cheek, "I personally believe there should only be two categories listed: 1) the baby won't come out (who knows why), and 2) the baby can't tolerate labor (i.e. distress). Maybe we could also add 3) maternal indications." How refreshingly clear and simple.

By contrast, in one National Center for Health Statistics document showing why cesareans were performed in 1992, there were fourteen medical risk factors listed, most involving health problems of the mother, plus fifteen additional complications that occur in labor and delivery. Another document from the same agency for the same year listed eight more complications. Among all of the complications, those with the word "labor" in their title included precipitous labor, prolonged labor, dysfunctional labor, seizures during labor, early or threatened labor, obstructed labor, and abnormal labor. Even if "dysfunctional" and "abnormal" mean the same thing, I had asked the obstetrician, what does "obstructed labor" mean? "These terms are very arbitrary," the obstetrician replied, followed by her preferred list of three categories.

Most of the indications doctors write on hospital charts do in fact fall into one of those three simple categories. It might be helpful to see whether the reasons your doctor gave for your first cesarean, fit into any of these. The obstetrician with the succinct definitions is my medical advisor for this book, Phyllis Marx, a

Chicago-area obstetrician. Her categories again: Was the baby simply not going to come out? Did labor pose a serious threat to the baby? Did the mother have a health problem, either unrelated or related to pregnancy, that made a cesarean safer than a vaginal birth? Your own answers to these questions may strongly affect how you feel now about that cesarean. Did the doctor explain to your satisfaction that it was the right thing to do, or do you suspect the doctor did it for reasons other than your benefit or the baby's? The answers to these questions will likely affect how you feel about attempting a trial of labor in your next pregnancy.

Though doctors can cite an almost infinite number of reasons for performing cesareans, more than 85 percent of those reasons fit into one of these four general groups: previous cesarean delivery (37.4 percent of all cesareans), dystocia (23.3 percent), breech presentation (14.7 percent), and fetal distress (10.3 percent).

Previous Cesarean Delivery

The single most common reason cesareans are performed is still because the mother had a previous cesarean. This reason definitely does not fit into one of Dr. Marx's three categories. While the fact that you had a prior cesarean may be a fine enough reason for you to have another one, it is no longer by itself considered a good medical reason.

In other words, if you had a low transverse uterine incision while undergoing one previous cesarean, that fact alone is not a medical reason for you to have a surgical delivery the next time. And some doctors go so far as to say that there is no reason why you should be allowed to have a surgical delivery until you have undergone labor and labor has failed. This is, of course, a controversial point in the cesarean debate.

Even the American College of Obstetricians and Gynecologists seems to contradict itself in the 1995 *ACOG Practice Patterns*, which contains clinical guidelines for VBAC. On the one hand, the document says, "Repeat cesarean births should not be done routinely, but rather for a specific indication." Two pages later, the

Table 3 Reasons for Cesareans (1993)

Category	Cesareans (Percent)
Repeat cesarean	37.4
Dystocia	
Prolonged labor	1.6
Dysfunctional labor	9.2
Cephalopelvic disproportion	12.5
Breech presentation	14.7
Fetal distress	10.3
Total of four categories	85.7

Source: National Center for Health Statistics. Monthly Vital Statistics Report; September 21, 1995; 44(35).

Note: These statistics are based on birth records (number of registered births), while the National Hospital Discharge Survey records (Tables 1 and 2) are based on deliveries reported by hospitals (not including military hospitals). Because the counting systems are different, the resultant numbers of total births, cesareans, and VBACs are different for each method, and the percentage rates are also slightly different. The National Center for Health Statistics advises using hospital data for long-term trends and registered births for one-year trends. The data in this table are based on 4,000,240 registered live births and 861,987 registered cesareans.

document states, "Actions or policies that coerce patients to undergo either a trial of labor or a repeat cesarean delivery interfere with patient autonomy and the informed consent process." The document tells physicians not to perform repeat cesareans routinely when there is no medical indication, but says if repeat cesarean is what the patient wants, the patient has the right to choose.

What does this really mean? Because of Craigin's dictum "Once a cesarean, always a cesarean," routine repeats were the rule as recently as fifteen years ago. But the incisions used in most cesareans today do not pose nearly the risk of rupture that the older style of incisions did. A repeat cesarean should no longer be done routinely, without discussion. Today, women have a choice of trying a vaginal delivery, and this choice should be discussed by doctor and patient. Then, after considering the option, if she still prefers to have a repeat cesarean, she should not be coerced into having a trial of labor. (That's what the document means to me, but not all doctors or insurers adhere to the part about choice.)

Forgetting for a moment how you feel about trying a vaginal delivery after a cesarean, look at how the people who want to lower the cesarean rate look at you, and why you are their top target. A national health objective is to lower the cesarean rate to 15 percent by the year 2000. Accomplishing that goal is contingent on increasing the VBAC rate to 35 percent. (Public Citizen, the consumer group founded by Ralph Nader, estimates the optimal VBAC rate to be 50 to 55 percent.) In 1992, if 35 percent of all women with a previous cesarean had delivered by VBAC, the overall cesarean rate would have been reduced from 22 percent to 18 percent. The increase in VBACs does contribute to the lowering of the cesarean rate, though it is certainly not the only factor.

The point of all these numbers is that the promotion of VBAC stems first and foremost from a national desire to lower the cesarean rate, which stems in turn from the drive to lower health care costs. Elective repeat cesareans are an easy target because there are a large number of them (336,000 in the United States in 1993) and the surgery is performed routinely, without determining whether it's medically necessary. The fact that the surgery is safe and often a more comfortable option for women who may have had a very rough first delivery seems to have been forgotten. The controversy over repeat cesareans is in small measure medical, in large measure economical. What is best for the economy, however, the least-expensive method, may or may not be what is best for you.

Dystocia

Dystocia is a catchall term that should probably be put to rest because it is vague and not easily understood. Second in frequency only to repeat cesarean, a diagnosis of dystocia accounts for 23.3 percent of all cesareans.

Dystocia means abnormally slow progress of labor. Exactly what *that* means, however, is open to interpretation. A true diagnosis of dystocia ultimately fits category number one above: the baby won't come out (who knows why). More specifically, a diagnosis of dystocia indicates one of several factors, including: involuntary uterine contractions aren't strong enough to dilate the cervix fully or to make the baby's presenting part descend; the voluntary pushing effort isn't strong enough once dilation is complete; there is a disproportion between the size of the baby's presenting part and the mother's pelvis that prevents the baby from getting out. Sometimes, a diagnosis of dystocia is a combination of these factors.

For instance, a woman can be experiencing strong uterine contractions that dilate her cervix to 4 centimeters, when contractions weaken, stalling the labor course; the cervix stops dilating and the baby does not descend. Or, a woman's cervix dilates all the way to 10 centimeters, but the baby hasn't descended. These scenarios can happen when part of the baby is too large to fit through the birth canal, or the chin isn't tucked into the chest, or the position of the head is slightly off. The cessation of normal labor, also called arrest of labor, may sometimes be a protective mechanism. A uterus typically does not keep contracting spontaneously with a strong enough force to lead to its rupture. An arrest of labor or an arrest of descent that does not respond to further standard interventions is a clear and necessary reason for a cesarean.

Scenarios like the one above happen frequently, but what's controversial is what doctors will or will not do to try to achieve a vaginal delivery, particularly in a woman giving birth for the first time. Perhaps the most common criticism of dystocia diagnoses results from a situation such as the following. A woman in her first pregnancy starts to have contractions, and she has them for many hours, perhaps even a day or longer; she comes to the hospital, exhausted, and she is only 3 centimeters dilated. The amniotic sac is still intact, and the baby is doing fine. A doctor who performs a cesarean at this stage can come under fire for not trying other measures.

One approach to this situation could be the old-fashioned nonmedical therapy of rest, patience, perhaps a warm bath if the amniotic sac is still intact, a soothing massage if desired, and maybe even a sedative to allow the mother to sleep through contractions. Of course, this lengthens the labor, and hospitals and doctors want to process women in and out as quickly as possible. A midwife, though, would be more likely to take this approach.

The other school of thought is to nudge things along by administering Pitocin (a synthetic form of the natural hormone, oxytocin) to strengthen contractions or by breaking the bag of waters. These interventions are part of a fairly recent concept called *active management of labor,* which was pioneered in Ireland in 1968 to control the cesarean rate and to give stalled labors an artificial jump-start. The use of active management of labor in the United States is increasing as hospitals try to reduce the number of cesareans performed for dystocia. Though the definition of the concept varies from institution to institution, there are generally several common components. The first is to establish a consistent definition for the symptoms that mark the actual onset of labor. The idea behind this is that if labor is diagnosed too early, interventions such as painkillers or epidurals may be given, which slow down the labor before it is well established. This is one reason books offering advice on how to avoid a cesarean encourage women to delay going to the hospital as long as they can, so as to avoid early interventions that may prolong labor.

In a study by José A. López-Zeno, M.D., conducted at Northwestern University in Chicago, comparing active management of labor with traditional management (the control group), spontaneous labor was defined as the presence of regular, painful contractions at least once every five minutes, as well as either complete effacement of the cervix or a broken amniotic sac.

The second component in the Northwestern study involved manually breaking the amniotic sac if it was still intact within one hour of the onset of spontaneous labor. Then, if the cervix dilated less than 1 centimeter per hour during the entire first stage (up until it was time to push), the progress was considered inadequate. Pitocin was then given at higher-than-usual doses to stimulate stronger contractions. Also, if the electronically monitored babies exhibited signs of fetal distress, fetal scalp samples were taken to test the pH of the babies' blood before doctors resorted to cesarean delivery.

A third, often unstated component of active management of labor is the setting of a twelve-hour time limit on the duration of labor. The idea is to deliver the baby within that time period, which means making every labor conform to a set of standards and employing Pitocin at a sufficient rate to achieve the goal. Depending on your view, this can be good or bad. Some women embrace the idea of having an endpoint in mind. Others want to give vaginal birth every possible chance, even if it takes three days.

In the Northwestern study, the cesarean rate in the actively managed group of 351 women was 10.4 percent, versus 14.1 percent in the traditionally managed group of 354 women. The authors reported no differences in the health of the babies, with slightly fewer infectious complications in the actively managed mothers. The labors of the active group averaged 6.5 hours from admission to delivery, as opposed to 8.2 hours for the control group.

The authors state that their definition of labor may prevent doctors from intervening *too* early, while conversely, the early use of Pitocin and breaking the sac could fix the sluggish uterine patterns before muscle fatigue sets in, thereby lowering the overall incidence of dysfunctional labor that leads to cesarean.

Using high doses of Pitocin is controversial, because it tends to produce overly strong uterine stimulation in half of all cases, which in turn can cause fetal distress, one of the other most common reasons for cesareans. Pitocin is not a gentle or pleasant drug—it makes contractions more intense and more painful—and its excessive use in VBAC patients as well as others is associated with increased complications for both babies and mothers. In one of the studies conducted by the Dublin, Ireland, group that originated the concept of active management of labor, the cesarean rate was very low in first-time mothers, just 5 percent, but not without considerable negative outcomes. A U.S. evaluation showed that the incidence of fetal deaths that occurred during labor in the Dublin hospital was seven times higher than in the Parkland Hospital in Dallas during the same time period, and the rate of neonatal seizures was twice as high. Furthermore, beyond what the term *active management* implies, there is a domino effect of interventions that tends to occur. While active management of labor may prevent cesareans and save money, it is hardly a process that allows birth to proceed on a natural course. For instance, Pitocin increases pain, which increases the desire for an epidural, which in turn can increase the likelihood of a forceps or cesarean delivery. On the other hand, judicious use of Pitocin and other interventions can in fact help prevent cesareans. Nobody can predict what will happen ahead of time, so it is important to be able to trust the decisions and skills of your caregiver.

If you are a VBAC candidate, and especially if the reasons for your first cesarean fall under the category of dystocia (see Chapter 3), you may want to think about the pros and cons of one surgical intervention, elective repeat cesarean, versus a possible host of interventions if your labor is actively managed.

Breech Birth

Cesareans performed because the baby is breech accounted for 14.7 percent of surgical deliveries in 1993. While breech babies in the past were frequently delivered vaginally, today about 85 percent of breeches are born by cesarean, because it is almost universally considered to be safer.

"The prognosis for the fetus in a breech presentation is considerably worse than when in a vertex [head down] presentation," write the authors of *Williams Obstetrics*. Breech babies tend to have slightly more abnormalities to begin with than vertex babies (the incidence of congenital abnormalities in one study was about 6.3 percent for babies who were breech at delivery versus 2.4 percent for vertex babies), but even when these are factored out, breech babies tend to suffer greater complications in vaginal delivery than vertex babies. However, cesarean delivery alone cannot assure a better fetal outcome.

The most common kind of breech is the frank breech, in which the buttocks, instead of the head, are the part of the baby born first (called the *presenting part*). A certain number of frank breech babies can be delivered vaginally. The second most common breech is the footling breech, in which one or both feet are the presenting part. According to *Williams Obstetrics,* numerous studies indicate that vaginal delivery of footling breeches at term is associated with "prohibitive perinatal mortality."

Why is vaginal delivery dangerous for breech babies? The most obvious reason is that the baby's head can get stuck in the birth canal after the buttocks or other parts have been delivered. This— along with the fact that the umbilical cord, containing the baby's blood supply, is pulled into the birth canal and becomes compressed —poses a danger of asphyxiation to the baby. Attempts to accelerate the delivery with forceps, especially in a footling breech, too often result in damage to the baby's brain, spinal cord, or skeleton.

The medical controversy isn't that a breech position is a bad reason to do a cesarean. What's controversial is that greater efforts are not being made to try to turn babies in utero so that they change from breech to the head-down position. If this procedure, called *external cephalic version,* were used more aggressively, critics of the high cesarean rate argue, perhaps 50 percent or more of the babies delivered by cesarean for breech presentation would be delivered vaginally. If this had been the case in 1992, it would have reduced the number of cesareans by 63,350.

External cephalic version, typically done after 37 weeks of gestation, also carries some risks (see Chapter 3). Though the likelihood of these risks occurring is low, they are significant and they include placental abruption (dislodging of the placenta, which nourishes the baby), uterine rupture, hemorrhage, preterm labor, and fetal distress requiring immediate cesarean delivery. Fetal death during version is not unheard of.

The use of version in VBAC candidates has not been proven safe, although a growing number of practitioners will try it in selected cases. When version doesn't work, or when the baby turns back to the breech position, should vaginal birth be attempted? Again, this is controversial. To assess the likelihood that the baby's head will pass through the pelvis, x-rays of the mother's pelvis may be taken to determine whether it is of normal size or unusually small. (However, such x-rays don't mean much without knowledge of the baby's size, which is why they have been abandoned for the most part.) Imaging of the baby is also needed to determine if the head is flexed (with the chin tucked into the chest) or extended (with the back of head bent toward the back). If the head is overly extended, vaginal breech delivery is unsafe.

According to clinicians discussing this issue in a roundtable symposium moderated by Jeffery P. Phelan, M.D. called "Finding Alternatives to Cesarean Section," the x-ray and sonogram tests eliminate about 50 percent of the breech babies as candidates for vaginal delivery.

Interestingly, the four male physicians at the symposium held contrasting views about the safety of vaginal breech deliveries, though all felt positive about version techniques. One doctor, Steven L. Clark, said that at his institution in Provo, Utah, vaginal breech deliveries were rare. "We've found that once a patient with a baby in breech position is truly informed regarding risks and benefits of a trial of labor, she will almost invariably choose the cesarean.

"I am reminded of a talk I gave to a group of physicians a few years ago," he continued. "I asked, 'How many of you allow a trial of labor in carefully selected patients with breech babies?' About two-thirds of the audience raised their hands. Then I said, 'How many would allow a trial of labor for your own child?' *None* of them raised their hands. I think the difference is that physicians are truly informed about the risks and benefits of the procedure in a way that patients—unless they're physicians them-selves—cannot be."

This anecdote is disturbing on several accounts. It implies that physicians who know full well the risks of a procedure are not communicating those risks sufficiently to their patients. It's like saying "What Mary doesn't know can't hurt her." It prevents the patient from making an informed choice. Dr. Clark's statement that patients cannot be fully informed unless they are physicians themselves may be true, but that does not excuse physicians from finding a way to explain such risks to the layperson. The anecdote also showed that physicians in that audience were comfortable with a lower standard of care for their patients than for their own loved ones. Would you willingly choose such a physician?

In sum, you should know that you don't have to try external cephalic version or vaginal breech delivery if you prefer not to.

Fetal Distress

Fetal distress is the primary reason listed for about 10 percent of cesareans in the United States. Proven fetal distress is a valid reason for performing a cesarean, and this diagnosis fits the category "the baby can't tolerate labor." But, like dystocia, the term fetal distress is too broad, and its diagnosis is often based on subjective judgments of fetal heart rate patterns. Some amount of stress accrues to the baby from the birth process itself. The challenge for the clinician is to separate the normal stresses of labor and delivery from stresses that could inflict lasting harm. This can be a difficult task. In part because of legal worries, some doctors may jump the gun and perform a cesarean prematurely, rather than risk further delay with a vaginal delivery. If you are the mother, are you more comfortable with the "better safe than sorry" approach, which results in cesarean delivery, or the more liberal "wait and see" approach, which may result in the vaginal delivery of an oxygen-deprived baby?

The incidence of fetal distress may be declining simply because the term is becoming so unpopular that doctors hesitate to use it. (It is not popular in medical legal circles either, because it leaves the caregiver open to accusations that something should have been done sooner to prevent damage that might have affected the baby.)

Instead, clinicians now are more inclined to say the heart rate patterns, based on fetal monitoring, were either *reassuring* or *nonreassuring*, which are more flexible and more fluid terms. A nonreassuring heart rate pattern doesn't necessarily mean the baby is in distress or needs to be delivered immediately, but it does mean continuous vigilance or further measures are necessary to see if the heart rate returns to expected levels.

Heart rate is complex and naturally variable from baby to baby, from the beginning to the end of one contraction, and from one stage of labor to the next (see Table 4, page 53). The most frequent cause for concern when the heart rate pattern looks abnormal is squeezing of the umbilical cord, which cuts off the baby's oxygen supply, usually temporarily. This can occur during a contraction or when the cord is wrapped tightly around some part of the baby. The baby's heart rate may decelerate, drop below the normal baseline (100 or 120 beats per minute) and rise again. Fetal bradycardia is a prolonged drop in the heart rate below the baseline. If it persists for five minutes, a cesarean may be in order.

Fetal tachycardia, a very rapid heartbeat, is usually a sign of stress, meaning that the baby's heart must work harder to extract oxygen. It can accompany maternal fever and the use of certain drugs. On the monitor, it is most nonreassuring if there is also decreased variability in the heart rate or late decelerations.

Before rushing to perform a cesarean, however, doctors can try other measures, such as changing the position of the mother, giving her oxygen in the hope that the baby will get more of it, and shutting off the Pitocin if it is being used. Also, taking a fetal scalp blood sample and measuring the pH of the baby's blood gives the most accurate assessment of whether the baby is or isn't getting enough oxygen. This test can only be done after the amniotic sac is broken. Most worrisome fetal heart rate patterns appear in the last two hours of labor, by which time the sac is usually broken anyway. More frequent use of fetal scalp sampling to confirm a suspected diagnosis of fetal distress has been called for because it is a reliable and low-risk measure that could help to lower the number of cesareans done for fetal distress.

Other Reasons for Cesareans

There are a multitude of other less common reasons for which cesareans are necessary.

Failed induction

Labor may be induced once you are approximately two weeks overdue, because the placenta may start to deteriorate and function less efficiently as pregnancy ends. Labor may be induced if you are diabetic, or have developed gestational diabetes, and the baby is expected to be large. Labor may be induced if you develop preeclampsia, a serious condition characterized by high blood pressure, excessive and sudden weight gain caused by fluid retention, and protein in the urine. If induction does not work in these cases, the baby must be delivered by cesarean.

Placenta previa

The placenta grows on the uterine wall during the first trimester of pregnancy. The developing fetus is attached to the placenta via the umbilical cord. The placenta functions as the vital go-between organ, carrying oxygen and nourishment from mother to baby, and taking carbon dioxide and other waste products from the baby back to the mother's blood supply, which can eliminate them. The placenta produces hormones to keep the uterine lining intact and to support the pregnancy, and it blocks some substances from reaching the baby while allowing others to cross. Normally, the placenta forms near the top or on the sides of the uterus. In placenta previa, it attaches to the uterus across the cervical opening, not only blocking the path of the baby but leaving the uterus vulnerable to excessive bleeding. Bleeding is usually the first symptom of placenta previa. The problem can also be diagnosed by ultrasound. Cesarean is the accepted method of delivery in this situation.

Placental abruption

Also called abruptio placenta, or premature separation of the placenta, abruption is the partial or total detachment of the placenta from the uterine wall during late pregnancy or labor. This puts both the baby and mother at great risk, and depending on the degree of the separation, a cesarean is usually required.

Umbilical cord prolapse

Occurring most often with breech births, prolapse of the umbilical cord is when the cord falls into the birth canal ahead of or along with the baby's presenting part. This is dangerous because the cord is very likely to get compressed, which shuts off the baby's oxygen supply and leads to severe fetal distress. A cesarean can save the baby's life.

Active genital herpes

A baby exposed to an active herpes infection in the birth canal can suffer life-threatening consequences. Rather than being too embarrassed to mention that you carry the herpes virus, it's a good idea to share this information with your doctor. If the infection isn't active, the baby won't contract it. But if even a mild outbreak has occurred close to your delivery, a cesarean can prevent the serious danger of exposure to the baby.

Multiple births

Mothers of twins and higher multiples tend to suffer greater than normal complications of pregnancy that may lead to cesarean. These include early labor, dysfunctional labor, umbilical cord prolapse, and early separation of the placenta, as well as unusual presentations, including twins that are joined (Siamese twins) or intertwined.

At least 50 percent of twin deliveries are cesareans. Twins tend to be premature and smaller than single babies, which puts them at greater risk for fetal distress. Occasionally, one twin will deliver vaginally, and one will have to be delivered by cesarean. Cesarean is usually performed if the first twin is not head down or if one is significantly larger than the other.

This is by no means a complete account of all the valid medical reasons for which cesareans are performed, just some of the more common ones. But if you are in doubt about the legitimacy of a planned cesarean you would rather avoid or a previous cesarean that seemed to proceed too hastily, remember the three simple categories. The baby wouldn't come out. The baby couldn't tolerate labor. You, the mother, had a complication that made cesarean safer than vaginal delivery. If the explanation you have been given does not fit one of these definitions, it may not be based on sound medical reasoning.

The Facts About VBAC

The national VBAC rate has risen astronomically in the past decade. In 1985, it was just 6.0 percent, and in 1988, 12.6 percent. Between 1988 and 1993, it more than doubled, to 25.4 percent. "VBAC rate" means, out of every 100 women with a prior cesarean section who gave birth again, 25.4 women had successful vaginal deliveries in 1993.

Another statistic you will hear when discussing VBAC with your doctor or midwife is that between 60 and 80 percent of women with a prior cesarean can safely delivery their next child vaginally. But if 60 to 80 percent of such women can have VBACs, you may ask, why is the VBAC rate still only 25.4 percent?

The 60 to 80 percent figures are taken from studies of women who actually attempted VBAC: of 100 women who, in physician lingo, "are allowed a trial of labor," 60 to 80 actually have vaginal births. But, in fact, only 40 to 50 out of 100 women with a previous cesarean are trying to have a VBAC. The simple explanation for why the VBAC rate isn't higher is because the number of women who are trying VBAC is relatively small. If only 40 women of 100 with a previous cesarean are trying to have a VBAC, and 60 percent of those succeed, the overall VBAC rate is 24 percent.

Why are only 40 to 50 out of 100 women with a previous cesarean trying VBAC? Here is where the statistics get confusing and difficult to interpret. One group of 100 urban women may have their babies in progressive teaching hospitals where VBACs are routinely offered and encouraged. A group of 100 rural women with fewer choices in providers and facilities may end up having their babies in small community hospitals that don't encourage or offer VBACs. It's certainly safe to say that not all eligible women are encouraged to try VBACs in the United States.

But there are other reasons the VBAC rate is not higher, not the least of which is that many women elect not to try it. According to the largest VBAC studies, in which VBAC has been actively encouraged, what the figure really means is that 50 to 60 percent of women are refusing to go through a trial of labor. In the largest U.S. VBAC studies to date, including a 5-year study by VBAC researcher Bruce Flamm, M.D., of 15,098 women in California with previous cesareans who were given the choice, only 5,733 women opted to try a VBAC, a total of 38 percent. (Usually, about 10 percent of women are found ineligible and excluded for such reasons as breech presentation, multiple fetuses, or gestational diabetes.) Since other VBAC studies show similar results— with only up to half of the women eligible for VBAC choosing to try it—it is safe to say that many women do not want VBACs.

At this writing, most women with a history of one or more cesareans may elect to have a repeat cesarean or to find a doctor who will grant this wish. But an alarming number of doctors, hospitals, insurance companies, and other policymakers are trying to take this choice away. Based on recent medical beliefs about the safety of VBAC—never mind its highly variable success rate—and based on the drive to lower medical costs, these powerful lobbies are moving in the direction of forcing women to have a trial of labor, whether they want to or not. The human element of giving birth, the unique concerns of a prior cesarean mother for her baby and herself, the fears that exist after a traumatic experience, are all cast aside. It's chilling to think that the history of women being told how to give birth is now continuing in another vein.

Who Can Attempt a VBAC?

The above notwithstanding, many women do prefer the VBAC option. If you are interested in having a VBAC, you will need to know the medical criteria that will be used to determine whether you are a good candidate.

The kind of incision you had is paramount. The vast majority of cesarean sections performed in the United States today are done with a low transverse uterine incision, the "bikini cut" across the abdomen just above the pubic bone. It is important to understand that the external skin incision may be different from the uterine incision. You could have an external horizontal incision, but a vertical uterine one. It is the uterine incision that matters in the next pregnancy.

Much rarer is the low vertical incision on the uterus. Vertical incisions are done when it is suspected that more room will be needed, so that the cut can be extended to a classical incision if necessary. Factors that may lead to this type of incision include extreme prematurity, placenta previa, or a transverse lie with the back down (the fetus is lying horizontally, face up, in the uterus).

The old-fashioned classical uterine incision is done in less than 10 percent of cesareans in the United States today. It is still done in other countries and also infrequently here when a woman goes into labor early with a very small baby or when the baby is transverse. In these cases, a classical incision makes it easier to get the baby out and is less traumatic to the baby.

If you had one previous low transverse incision, the *1995 ACOG Practice Patterns* guidelines recommend to physicians that you should be "counseled and encouraged to undergo a trial of labor" in your current pregnancy, unless you have contraindications.

If you have had more than one cesarean with a low transverse incision, most studies indicate that the risks to you and your baby are no greater than for women with one prior cesarean. The guidelines advocate a trial of labor for "selected women" in this group, so this is something to discuss in depth with your doctor. The guidelines say there is not enough data to make a recommendation for women who have had a low vertical incision, or for women who have had a myomectomy (removal of a fibroid tumor).

If you meet the stated criteria, the guidelines further recommend that a trial of labor and delivery occur in a hospital setting that has the resources to respond to acute intrapartum (during labor) obstetric emergencies. The most serious medical risk of VBAC to both the mother and baby is a complete rupture of the uterus at the scar site. If this happens, the baby must be delivered immediately by cesarean section because blood flow to the baby may be compromised. Unfortunately, if the rupture is discovered too late, the baby or mother may die. Immediate measures must also be taken to repair the mother's uterus and prevent excessive blood loss. In some cases, a hysterectomy is necessary because the uterus can't be saved. The risk of uterine rupture in women with low incisions who attempt VBAC is less than 1 percent. However, the ACOG guidelines recommend that a "physician who is capable of evaluating labor, performing a cesarean delivery, and managing the complications of uterine rupture should be readily available."

A less serious risk of VBAC is a separation or tear in the uterine scar, which occurs in up to 2 percent of women with low transverse incisions. These tears may be asymptomatic, without pain or bleeding, and are usually only discovered during an exam after the VBAC. Though they heal by themselves, there is little if any data on the risks such tears may pose for future pregnancies.

If you or your doctor suspect you are carrying a large baby, defined by ACOG as weighing more than 4000 grams (8 lbs. 13 oz.), this factor alone should not preclude you from attempting VBAC if you want to. However, the larger the baby, the less likely the VBAC will succeed.

A 1989 study by Bruce Flamm looked at the percentages of women who were able to have a VBAC in relation to the birthweight of the baby. In the largest group, with babies weighing less than 4000 grams (8 lbs. 13 oz.), 78 percent of 1475 women who attempted VBAC succeeded. In the second group, with babies weighing between 4000 and 4499 grams (8 lbs. 13 oz. to 9 lbs. 14 oz.), 58 percent of 240 women had successful vaginal deliveries. In the third group, with babies weighing 4500 grams or more (9 lbs. 15 oz. and up), only 43 percent of 61 women were able to deliver vaginally.

Despite his own data, Dr. Flamm concludes that the medical literature "does not support elective cesarean section for suspected fetal macrosomia [large body] in non-diabetic women." Even if you have just a 43 percent chance, or a 58 percent chance, of a successful VBAC, he says he would not support elective cesarean in your circumstances because fetal macrosomia cannot be reliably predicted in advance by current clinical methods. Ultrasound measurements can be way off, especially as the baby gets large. In fact, studies have shown that women are more often correct than physicians in predicting their baby's birthweight.

It is interesting to note that the overall VBAC rate in the same study in 301 women with babies weighing 4000 grams or more was only 55 percent, while the vaginal delivery rate in a control group of 301 women with large babies but no previous cesarean section was 89 percent. The authors offer no explanation for this difference, nor do they include the reasons for the primary cesareans in the first group. One possibility is that some of these women were unable to deliver large babies vaginally before and that the same thing has happened in the subsequent birth.

One thing you are sure to hear from pro-VBAC practitioners is that they have delivered VBAC babies that are considerably larger than the mothers' previous cesarean baby. In some cases, the position of the cesarean baby in the birth canal has more bearing on the outcome than the size. But someone who dismisses the baby's size or says it has no bearing on the likelihood of a successful VBAC is not telling the whole truth.

Who Shouldn't Attempt a VBAC?

The 1994 ACOG VBAC guidelines (a more general document than *ACOG Practice Patterns*) consider a previous classical uterine incision a contraindication to a trial of labor. Women with such an incision, says ACOG, "should be strongly discouraged" because this type of incision is associated with a uterine rupture rate of up to 12 percent.

Not enough is known yet to assess the safety of labor after cesarean in women carrying more than one fetus, according to ACOG.

The safety of VBAC can also not be determined in women with breech babies (when the buttocks or feet are positioned to come out first), according to ACOG, because only a small number of such patients have been studied. But the issue is neverthe-less controversial. In 1993, according to the National Center for Health Statistics, 85.2 percent of breech babies were delivered by cesarean, and a breech presentation accounted for 14.7 percent of all cesarean deliveries.

In *Unnecessary Cesarean Sections*, the authors argue in favor of greater use of external cephalic version, a method of manually turning the fetus to the head-down position after the 37th week of pregnancy. The procedure requires that the mother be medi-cated and, since complications can occur involving the umbilical cord and the placenta (in about 1.5 percent of cases), it needs to be done in a hospital with an ultrasound and where immediate cesarean section is available. Studies show that the procedure is successful 48 to 77 percent of the time, but 2.5 percent of suc-cessfully turned babies may turn back again. There is limited data on whether external cephalic version can be done safely and suc-cessfully in women with a previous cesarean.

Other contraindications for a trial of labor after a cesarean are the same as those that precluded labor for a primary cesarean, and even these are controversial. Depending on your physician, these may include predetermined fetal distress, hypertension (high blood pressure), diabetes or gestational diabetes, genital herpes, eclampsia, hydramnios or oligohydramnios (too much or not enough amniotic fluid). Most primary cesareans are done, however, after labor has begun, some complication arises, and the baby won't come out. Common diagnoses include cephalopelvic disproportion (the baby is too large or the pelvis is too small for the baby to fit through the birth canal), fetal distress (the baby's heart rate pattern indicates that oxygen flow may be compromised), and arrest of labor (dila-tion or descent stops, even though contractions may continue).

Since these problems are generally not predictable in advance, VBAC advocates argue that any probability of their reoccurring should be ignored. The risk, of course, is that they will reoccur and that you will go through another labor and end up with a cesarean section once again. All but a few studies have ignored the effect such an experience, or even the fear of such an experi-ence, may have on women.

Are There Predictors of Success?

The likelihood you will succeed at VBAC if you are deemed medically eligible and if you try it is between 60 and 80 percent. Let's say it's 70 percent, halfway between those two numbers. But for you it will be either 0 or 100 percent. How will you know if you will fall into the lucky 70 percent group, or the other 30 percent category, the ones who go through labor and end up with a repeat cesarean?

A few studies have tried to determine if there are certain predictors of success. Success is medically defined as vaginal delivery of a live infant. "Success" is a bare-bones option—it does not come with any guarantees about the quality of the experience, such as the length of labor, the amount of pain, the use of drugs to induce or augment labor, the use of forceps or vacuum extractor, or the cutting of an episiotomy. Any combination of these that results in a live birth, regardless of your comfort level with them, constitutes a "success" in medical terms.

One potentially promising procedure for determining whether your baby will fit through your birth canal is a measurement called the *fetal-pelvic index*. Instead of relying only on ultrasound estimates of the baby's weight near birth, which have a high rate of error and which can't take the mother's pelvis into account, this technique literally measures the size of the passenger (fetus) versus the size of the passage (pelvis). Ultrasound measurements are taken of the circumference of the baby's head and abdomen, which tend to be more predictive than weight estimates. These are compared with x-ray measurements of the mother's pelvic inlet and midpelvic diameters. When the fetal-pelvic index is positive, the baby's measurements are too big for the mother's, and the baby won't fit. When it is zero or negative, the baby will fit. If the baby is lying in an occiputposterior position, meaning the back of its head is hitting against the mother's sacrum—which results in exceptionally painful back labor—the index must be more negative, –6 or lower, for the baby to fit through the mother's pelvis.

In clinical trials, the index has compared very favorably with either of the traditional methods used alone (ultrasound estimates of fetal birthweight and x-ray measures of the pelvis). Studied now for about ten years, most extensively by doctors at the University of Oklahoma College of Medicine in Oklahoma City, it has proven to be highly predictive. It is simple to administer and inexpensive. In a recent study by Gary Thurnau, M.D., in the *American Journal of Obstetrics and Gynecology*, 13 VBAC candidates with a positive index all ended up with a repeat cesarean, while 47 VBAC candidates with a negative index all ended up with a vaginal delivery.

What appears to be controversial about this method, from a consumer's point of view, is the taking of an x-ray of the pregnant mother's pelvis near delivery. (Ultrasound cannot be used because it measures soft tissue, not bone.) If you are old enough, you may remember that pregnant women's pelvises used to be x-rayed years

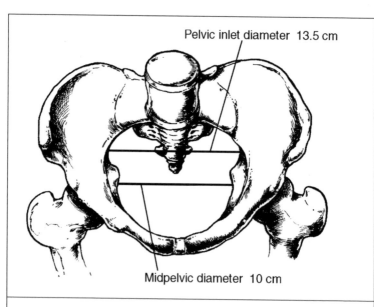

Pelvic inlet diameter 13.5 cm

Midpelvic diameter 10 cm

Pelvic Measurements and the Fetal-Pelvic Index

Measurements of the fetal-pelvic index, which can determine whether a baby will fit through a pelvis, take four pelvic diameters into account, including the two transverse (across) diameters shown here: the pelvic inlet and the midpelvic diameters. Note the ischial spines, the two bony protrusions marking the midpelvic diameter.

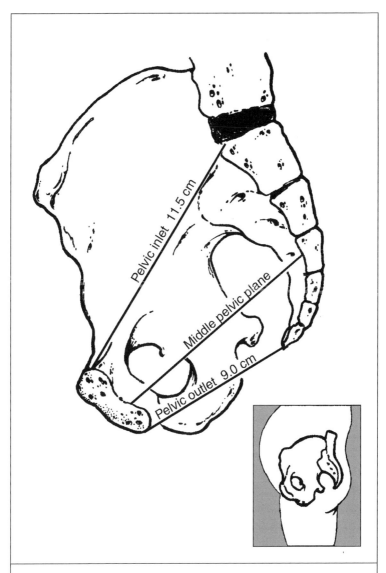

The two upper diameters shown here, the pelvic inlet and mid-pelvic plane, measure the pelvis from front to back. (The pelvic outlet, though narrower than the midpelvic plane, tends to stretch more.) To obtain the fetal-pelvic index, the circumferences of the inlet and middle plane are determined by taking the average of the two pelvic inlet diameters and the average of the two midpelvic diameters and multiplying each by 3.142.

ago, but the practice fell out of favor. According to Dr. Thurnau, x-rays fell out of favor primarily because they were not very useful, and on top of that, there was some concern about radiation to the fetus. Dr. Thurnau says the amount of radiation transmitted to the fetus in his studies, between 80 and 1000 millirads, is far below the 15-rad danger zone (1000 millirads = 1 rad) and sufficiently below the 5-to-10 rad gray zone (questionable zone). The

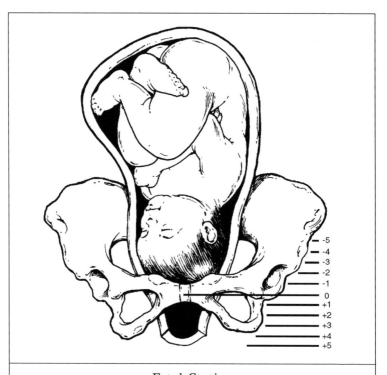

Fetal Station

At –5, the baby's head has not entered the pelvis; it is still above the pelvic inlet. At 0, the presenting part of the baby (ideally, the head) is at the level of the ischial spines, meaning that the widest part of the head has reached the narrowest part of the pelvis. Once the head has passed 0, the baby has an excellent chance of delivering vaginally. At +5, the baby's head is starting to crown. Since each station is only 1 centimeter from the next—the total range of distance is just 10 centimeters (4 inches)—and since the stations are not measured but estimated manually, error can easily be introduced.

risk of childhood leukemia after exposure to x-rays in utero has been measured as 1 in 2000, compared with 1 in 2880 in unirradiated children. This risk is considered insignificant, especially because the incidence of childhood leukemia is already low.

Unfortunately, Dr. Thurnau's work has not been duplicated in other institutions, for several reasons, including the fact that x-ray pelvimetry is no longer used in most institutions. A CT scan of the mother's pelvis is equally reliable and transmits less radiation. Magnetic resonance imaging (MRI) would be a good substitute for x-rays because it does not irradiate at all, but it is very expensive.

"My personal bias is that the fetal-pelvic index would help a great deal," says Watson Bowes, M.D., professor of obstetrics and gynecology at the University of North Carolina in Chapel Hill, an institution that lobbied unsuccessfully for funding of a pilot study on the index. "But corroborative studies need to be done before we can be really enthusiastic. On the other hand, if a practitioner read the papers on the index and offered the test as a way to help make a decision and did it with the full informed consent of the patient, I don't think it would be unethical. The patient would know the risks and benefits and could decide whether to have the test done."

In 1993, a diagnosis of cephalopelvic (also called fetopelvic) disproportion was listed as a complication in 110,076 live births, and 97.6 percent of these were delivered by cesarean section. When taking all 861,987 cesareans into account for 1993, 12.5 percent were attributed to cephalopelvic disproportion. But the real number may be greater because big babies that get stuck in narrow passages may also account for some of the diagnoses of abnormal or dysfunctional labor, prolonged labor, and fetal distress.

The term dystocia, which has recently fallen out of favor because of its vagueness, used to include any diagnosis of abnormal labor. In 1993, dystocia was the second most commonly cited reason for cesarean section (23.3 percent of the total, behind repeat cesarean, 37.4 percent). A substantial number of these dystocia diagnoses are possibly due to big babies that will not fit.

A safe and accurate way of determining which babies would fit and which wouldn't could be quite important to women interested in VBAC. First, an accurate assessment of the baby-to-mother fit would give both mothers and doctors more objective and individualized data than is currently available for determining the chances of success. Why there is no such test available now is perplexing, since there is clearly a need. Perhaps a lot more than 50 to 60 percent of women eligible for VBAC would opt for a trial of labor if they believed it would really work *for them.* Second, it would save a lot of wasted time, both for the women who could avoid a long unproductive labor and for the attendants who stand by waiting. Third, though cost should not be the decisive issue when it comes to childbirth, foregoing ten, twenty, or more pointless hours in hospital-room costs each time a trial of labor fails could amount to substantial savings. Furthermore, complications are greater in women who have a non-elective or emergency cesarean than in women who have an elective cesarean, and recovery times for the former are longer.

A few other studies have looked for clues for predicting whether a VBAC would succeed. A 1988 study by David Ollendorff, M.D., at Northwestern University Medical School looked for a relationship between how much a woman had dilated in her cesarean labor and her chances of success at VBAC, but found none. The study did find a big difference in outcomes based on birthweight: the VBAC rate for mothers giving birth to babies weighing less than 4000 grams (8 lbs. 13 oz.) was 81 percent, versus only 40 percent for babies weighing 4000 grams or more.

An interesting study by Lisa R. Troyer, M.D., at the University of Texas Health Science Center in Houston looked retrospectively at a group of 264 women who labored after a cesarean, of whom 192, or 72.7 percent, delivered vaginally. The researchers identified four risk factors that lowered the VBAC rate and assigned each a point value of 1. In order of their significance, the risk factors were nonreassuring fetal heart tracing on admission (an indication of fetal distress), induction of labor, previous dysfunctional labor (including failure to progress and cephalopelvic disproportion), and no prior vaginal delivery. Of the women with a score of 0, or no risk factors, 91.5 percent had successful VBACs. Women with scores of 1, 2, and 3 had VBAC rates of

73.9 percent, 66.7 percent, and 50 percent respectively. Only two women had a score of 4, and both required a cesarean section. However, as the authors point out, two is too small a number on which to base conclusions. Furthermore, retrospective studies can't be predictive; you can't tell ahead of time whether induction of labor will become necessary or if fetal distress will occur. But the study suggests that if your labor is induced in a VBAC attempt or if you had dysfunctional labor before, your chances of a successful VBAC may be reduced.

Finally, a pair of investigators in New York, led by Mortimer G. Rosen, M.D., did what is called a meta-analysis of twenty-nine individual studies on indicators of successful VBAC. From all the studies analyzed together, they came to the following conclusions:

- Women who had a cesarean for a breech delivery had twice the success rate at VBAC of women whose cesarean was done for other reasons. (This implies that the complication of a breech position is a lot less likely to reoccur than other complications.)

- Women with a previous vaginal delivery had twice the success rate at VBAC than women without one.

- Women whose previous cesarean was for cephalopelvic disproportion were only half as likely to succeed as women whose previous cesarean was done for other reasons. (In other words, cephalopelvic disproportion is more likely to reoccur than other complications.)

- Women who were given Pitocin to increase contractions during a trial of labor had only one third the chance of successful VBAC as women who did not receive Pitocin.

- Women with more than one previous cesarean were only two thirds as likely to succeed as women with only one previous cesarean.

When I was deemed a good VBAC candidate for the birth of my second son in 1992, the only statistical information I was given was the overall success rate of 60 to 80 percent of those who try. I didn't think the numbers were particularly wonderful—a grade of 60 on an exam amounts to a D. And I wondered even then how well the numbers spoke to my specific situation. Had I known then what I know now—that my chances were really closer to 40 to 60 percent because of the reasons for my primary cesarean (my first baby had weighed 9 lbs. 13 oz., I experienced arrest of labor for four hours, and I was given Pitocin with negligible results)—I might have trusted more in my own instincts, which told me I was not in fact a great candidate for VBAC.

Statistics and studies are of vital concern to the scientific and medical communities and to patients. But statistics are impersonal, and they are ultimately only helpful if they apply when it's your baby. It might be useful to explore the topic in more depth with your doctor if you have unique concerns that are not addressed by the 60-to-80-percent figure. You may want to ask for more detail on issues like cephalopelvic disproportion, failure to progress, or induction of labor. If your doctor doesn't seem interested in the reasons for your previous cesarean (which may be the case if it's a different doctor), that should be a red flag.

When Are You Most Likely to Have a VBAC?

Apart from your doctor's influence and your own medical history, other nonmedical factors will have a bearing on your journey through the medical maze. Your age, level of education, socioeconomic status, and ethnic makeup may affect the likelihood of your having a VBAC. Additionally, the kind of insurance you have, where you live, and certain characteristics of the hospital where you deliver all have an effect on the outcome.

In a recent *Journal of the American Medical Association* article (August 94), researchers Dale E. King, M.A., and Kajal Lahiri, Ph.D., analyzed 13,944 births in 1989 to women in New York State with a history of cesarean delivery. The overall VBAC rate was 22 percent. Women with 17 or more years of education had the highest VBAC rate (28.6 percent), followed by women with 16 years

(24.8 percent), down to women with less than 12 years, who had the lowest rate (19.2 percent).

However, looking at vital statistics from the same year in New York, the researchers found that women with 17 or more years of education also had the highest first cesarean rate (17.5 percent), while those with less than 12 years had the lowest (13.2 percent). The authors, who are not physicians, speculate that the discrepancy may be because many women are unhappy with their first cesarean and the more educated women are more proactive in seeking out the VBAC alternative for their next delivery. A separate editorial in *JAMA* by ACOG executive director Ralph Hale, M.D., challenges this assumption, saying it "ignores the positive reasons for a cesarean delivery, which in many instances is well accepted by the patient, especially when it saves the life of her child or allows her to give birth to an otherwise undeliverable infant." Maybe the women with the most education are simply getting the most appropriate care, with both the higher primary cesarean rate and the higher VBAC rate being justified. As the editorial points out, since the researchers did not have the data explaining the reasons for the primary cesarean and since they could not tell whether there was a failed trial of labor in the VBAC attempt, it's hard to draw conclusions based on level of education alone.

The researchers also found that the odds of VBAC increased with the level of care provided by the hospital. Hospitals with intensive neonatal care facilities (also called level 3 or tertiary care hospitals) had the highest rate of VBAC, which is consistent with the findings of other studies. Teaching hospitals had the highest VBAC rate and government hospitals had the lowest, also consistent with other findings. Women insured by HMOs were more likely to have VBAC than women with private insurance. Interestingly, white women had higher VBAC rates than either African American or Hispanic women, but other nonwhite women (including Asian women) had the highest VBAC rate of all (29.4 percent).

A California study by Randall S. Stafford, Ph.D., of 45,425 births to women with a previous cesarean (for an overall VBAC rate of 10.9 percent in 1986 looked separately at age, race, socioeconomic status, and hospital characteristics. Women under 25 had a higher VBAC rate than women over 35, and white women had a higher rate than African American and Hispanic women.

Women of higher socioeconomic status had a lower VBAC rate, or higher repeat cesarean rate. The researchers attribute this finding to the differences in hospital settings in which wealthy versus indigent women are likely to give birth, rather than to a difference in the way physicians might treat these two groups.

However, the finding that women of higher socioeconomic status have lower VBAC rates (and higher overall cesarean rates) is consistent with other studies, and it raises some interesting questions. One of the biggest issues confronting our health care system today is the discrepancy between care for the poor and uninsured versus care for the more fortunate and well-insured. While HMOs appear to be the wave of the future, they have come under widespread attack for not ensuring the quality of care that private insurance provides. It is not unreasonable to wonder whether many lesser-insured and indigent women are having more VBACs because they cost less, and because poor women are less likely to have a voice in the decision than affluent women.

In a chilling *New York Times* series in March 1995 investigating the reasons for higher infant mortality rates in public hospitals (which serve indigent people) than private ones, the paper cited numerous examples of women whose babies died or were permanently damaged because no qualified physicians were present to perform a lifesaving cesarean. In a short article called "Too Few Cesareans?" the *Times* noted that the percentage of cesareans performed in cases of fetal distress, in which the baby is deprived of oxygen, was only 26.8 percent at North Central Bronx versus 60.9 percent in the city's private hospitals.

The *Times* series did not look at VBAC rates; however, as the title of the article above suggests, when the system cracks and medical resources are stretched too thin, indigent women and their babies are the first to suffer. In case after case in the *Times* series, poor women who should have received a cesarean didn't. If affluent women are getting more cesareans, maybe there are valid reasons. If the contrast in New York City between public and private care is a microcosm of how the rest of the system functions, it may be just as important to ask if indigent women and their babies are being deprived of needed cesareans as it is to suggest that affluent women are getting too many.

The California study also found that private hospitals had the lowest VBAC rates; the University of California, a public facility, had the highest. Privately insured women had the lowest VBAC rates, while those insured by Kaiser Permanente, a large pro-VBAC HMO, had the highest. VBAC rates were three times higher in high-volume hospitals than in low-volume hospitals.

A Canadian study by Gail Goldman, B.Sc., of Quebec women who gave birth between 1985 and 1988 found that women were more likely to have a VBAC if their doctor was younger than 54, if his or her cesarean rate was less than 20 percent, and if less than 5 percent of his patients were considered high risk. Patients with a lower level of education had a higher VBAC rate than better-educated patients, a finding that conflicts with the New York State data.

If you feel strongly about wanting a VBAC, consider all of the above and figure out what you can and can't control. Obviously, you can't control your age or race. Your level of education and socioeconomic status may or may not change during your child-bearing years. You may not be able to switch the type of insurance coverage you have. But if you have private insurance and even if you have HMO insurance, you still have important choices: your selection of a physician or midwife and the setting in which you will deliver (see Chapter 6).

These two players—physician or caregiver, and hospital—are key. Your medical history is important, but it may be interpreted differently by two different caregivers. How do you interpret your medical history? Do you think your first cesarean was necessary or reasonable, or could you have labored longer and delivered vaginally? Do you think it's likely the same complications could arise again, or was the first situation unique? What kind of birth do you think you would be most comfortable with? Do you want to get it over with as quickly as possible, or are you excited about experiencing the natural process of giving birth? You are the mother-to-be, the one carrying the child, the one who must advocate for this child and for yourself. Don't underestimate your strongest playing card: you. The more informed, empowered, and assertive you are in exercising as much choice as you can, the more likely you are to have the kind of experience you want.

How Is VBAC Different
from Routine Vaginal Birth?

The main difference between the way the physician, hospital, and attending staff handle you when you are trying to have a VBAC from the way they would treat someone without a previous cesarean is to have a heightened awareness of the possibility of uterine rupture. If you are in a hospital, you will be hooked up to an electronic fetal monitor, as you probably were before. One of the two straps wrapped around your abdomen picks up the baby's heart rate via ultrasound. The other is a pressure-sensitive device that detects the timing and strength of your uterine contractions. At first you and the baby will be monitored externally. After the amniotic sac is broken, an internal monitor may be attached to the baby's scalp.

You can watch the machine graph out the two measurements on the roll of paper and see the next contraction coming before you feel it (and see relief in sight when the line drops down). The printout can be especially useful if your contractions are regular, as it can help you establish a rhythm and prepare yourself for what's to come.

The fetal heart rate should hover between 120 and 160 beats per minute, but sometimes it may drop below that. There is cause for concern when the fetal heart rate stays low for prolonged periods, as the baby may not be getting enough oxygen, a sign of fetal distress. Electronic fetal monitors are the modern way of diagnosing fetal distress, but they are controversial (see Chapter 1), not because they cause harm to either mother or baby, but because they have been blamed for promoting needless cesarean sections. Also, as long as you are hooked up to the monitor, your movement is restricted. However, in most cases, a woman doesn't need to be hooked up continuously, especially during early labor when it may be more productive to walk and move if possible. And some hospitals have portable monitors that allow you to walk.

ACOG recommends that VBAC candidates need not be restricted to a labor bed before active labor has begun. Active labor is the phase when the cervix is between 4 and 7 centimeters dilated. Contractions occur every two to five minutes and last about sixty seconds.

For women attempting a VBAC, the monitor should be closely watched for signs of uterine rupture, especially as labor progresses. (Since it should be closely and regularly watched in all labors for signs of fetal distress, some physicians say management of a VBAC labor is really no different.) The signs of uterine rupture include a sudden change in fetal heart rate and a sudden change in uterine activity or pressure, both of which are most rapidly detected by the electronic monitor. Other signs include vaginal bleeding, a loss of fetal station (a number between −5 and +5 designating the position of the baby's head in the pelvis), and a severe pain that persists even when contractions are over.

There are not any other predetermined differences between the management of a routine vaginal birth and a VBAC. ACOG recommends that if you are planning a VBAC, your trial of labor and delivery should "occur in a hospital setting that has the professional resources to respond to acute intrapartum obstetric emergencies," and that "a physician who is capable of evaluating labor and performing a cesarean delivery should be readily available." However, contrary to a statement in the 1991 revised and expanded edition of the popular pregnancy book *What to Expect When You're Expecting*, "If you are to succeed at VBAC, you will need to find an amenable doctor who is willing to be with you from the beginning of labor through delivery," don't count on the presence of your doctor, no matter how amenable she is, from beginning to end. Finding a doctor who can or will commit to that amount of time would be the exception rather than the rule. However, the idea that you could use some extra support is a very sound one (see Chapter 5, page 103) that doesn't get a lot of airing in U.S. medical journals but is a popular practice in foreign countries. If you feel the need for extra support and expertise during labor, you may want to invest a couple of hundred dollars to hire a qualified birth attendant, also called a *doula* or *monitrice,* in addition to the emotional support you will need from a husband or trusted partner.

A lot of women wonder whether they can have an epidural during a VBAC. The answer is a resounding yes. "Contemporary experience suggests that the use of epidural analgesia neither delays the diagnosis of uterine rupture nor decreases the likelihood of a successful trial of labor," state the 1994 ACOG guidelines. Further, the same document says, "the availability and use of epidural analgesia probably encourages a greater percentage of women to choose a trial of labor."

If you are considering selecting a midwife as your provider, be sure to discuss this topic ahead of time if it's important to you. Many midwives shun epidurals in the belief that they inhibit labor, interfere with pushing, and initiate a cascade of additional interventions, thereby increasing the likelihood of cesarean delivery. One Chicago midwife I interviewed said she would not agree ahead of time to let a VBAC candidate have an epidural, and would only do so if and when she (the midwife) deemed it appropriate and absolutely necessary.

Despite the anti-epidural sentiment of many midwives, the specific combination of drugs in epidurals has improved in recent years (though not necessarily universally), and many women report being able to push adequately and forcefully while still experiencing pain relief from an epidural.

You may also wonder about the use of Pitocin during a VBAC labor and whether it's safe, since it increases the power of contractions. Pitocin is definitely used by doctors and sometimes by midwives in much the same way it would be used in a routine vaginal delivery, to try to produce stronger, more effective contractions when cervical dilation slows or stops. While Pitocin should not be used in a woman with a classical incision, according to ACOG (and ACOG says such a woman should not be laboring anyway), its careful, appropriate use does not confer a greater risk to a laboring woman with a low incision, nor is it

Table 4 Stages and Phases of Labor			
Stage	Phase	Frequency/ Length of Contractions	What Happens
First			Contractions; possible "lightening" feeling as the baby's position drops; cervix dilates to 10 cm
	Latent	As far apart as every 30 min. to as close as every 5 min./ As short as 10 sec. to as long as 60 sec.	Cervix dilates to 3 to 4 cm
	Active	Every 5 min. to every 2 min. / 60 sec.	Cervix dilates from 4 cm to 7 cm
	Transition	Every 1 min. to 3 min. / 60 to 90 sec.	Cervix dilates from 7 cm to 10 cm
Second			Urge to push; birth of baby
Third			Delivery of the placenta

Note: This is roughly the course of labor in an uncomplicated vaginal delivery.

associated with increased infant death rates. Less is known about *inducing* labor with Pitocin and making the cervix more favorable with prostaglandin gel, according to ACOG, although some hospitals use these methods routinely.

Studies (such as the aforementioned Houston study) report a lower rate of VBAC success in women whose labor is induced, and unless the baby is late and thought to be quite large or unless there is another reason to get it out pronto, most doctors and midwives prefer to let labor begin on its own. However, if you are interested in a VBAC but past your due date, and you have reason to believe you are carrying a large baby (perhaps your cesarean involved a baby that wouldn't fit), induction of labor is definitely worth discussing.

You may also justifiably wonder if your labor with a VBAC will last as long as the labor that ended with a cesarean. *What to Expect When You're Expecting* says that "your labor this time is likely to be much easier and shorter." However, two 1990 studies published in *Obstetrics and Gynecology* indicate that this is untrue. In women whose primary section was for labor abnormalities and who had had no prior vaginal birth, the trial of labor in the VBAC attempt was similar in length or longer than a first labor. In one of the studies, women whose cesarean was performed in the latent phase of labor (less than 4 centimeters dilated) had longer subsequent labors than women laboring for the first time. Sectioned women with a previous vaginal birth labored similarly to nonsectioned women with a previous vaginal birth.

These studies were not done to help you decide whether you want a trial of labor but to help obstetricians "revise their expectations and not anticipate that these individuals will progress as rapidly in labor as women who previously had vaginal deliveries," according to Frederick E. Harlass, M.D., author of one of the studies. (And don't expect a pro-VBAC doctor to revise *your* expectations by volunteering this information.) The authors of the other study, Cynthia Chazotte, M.D., Robert Madden, Ph.D., and Wayne R. Cohen, M.D., write that if physicians anticipate a VBAC labor that is similar in duration to a first labor, they will be less likely to overdiagnose labor abnormalities and less likely to perform unnecessary repeat cesareans.

If you are committed to trying VBAC, it may help to be prepared for a long labor. Then, if it's natural and swift, you'll be happily surprised. If you are uncertain about attempting a trial of labor, you have good reason to be—there are many unknowns. If it's okay for doctors to be equivocal and tell you that you have a 70 percent chance of success at VBAC, it's okay for you to be equivocal about your decision. All you can do is make the best possible judgment about your own chances of success. It is important, too, to trust your instincts and feelings. If you are convinced that VBAC won't work, there's no point forcing yourself to go through with it.

FOUR

· · · · ·

Weighing the Risks

When you are trying to decide between a repeat cesarean and an attempted vaginal delivery, you need to know the medical risks of each method to yourself and your baby. If you searched the medical literature, you would find numerous papers and studies testifying that VBAC is safer than elective repeat cesarean, and others that cast some doubt. If there is any consensus, it would seem to be that VBAC may be slightly safer for the mother, while elective repeat cesarean may be slightly safer for the baby.

"If you do a VBAC, you put the risk on the child," says Leslie Iffy, M.D., professor of obstetrics and gynecology at the New Jersey Medical School in Newark. "If you do a cesarean section, you put the risk on yourself."

The good news is that the safety differences are relatively small. Both methods are statistically very safe for you and your baby when your health is good and when you receive good obstetrical care throughout pregnancy and delivery. The hard part is that you and your doctor still have to choose which method is best for you.

The comparison between VBAC and elective repeat cesarean is not the same as that between a first vaginal birth and a first cesarean, especially if the first cesarean occurred after labor, under urgent circumstances. A planned elective repeat cesarean is less risky than an emergency cesarean performed to save the baby after the mother has labored to exhaustion. On the other hand, if your first cesarean was scheduled and you didn't labor, you experienced something similar to an elective repeat cesarean. A trial of labor after a cesarean carries greater risks than a vaginal delivery in someone with no uterine scar.

What you really have to compare are the risks of three scenarios: elective repeat cesarean, a successful vaginal delivery after cesarean, and an attempted vaginal delivery that ends in another cesarean. Elective repeat cesarean means you have scheduled surgery with no labor. A successful VBAC means that you labor and give birth without surgery. An attempted vaginal delivery that ends in another cesarean—doctors call this a failed trial of labor—means that first you labor, then have another unscheduled surgery. In all three scenarios, you will be contending with the uterine scar from your previous operation.

Let's start with what physicians seem to agree about. Now that VBAC has been offered on a large scale in the United States for more than a decade, most physicians would agree that a trial of labor is safe in a woman with one low transverse uterine incision who is carrying one fetus in a head-down position and who has no other contraindications (such as genital herpes), *as long as she is closely monitored in labor.*

Most physicians would also agree that an elective repeat cesarean is a relatively safe operation. Medical advances in anesthesia, surgical techniques, the handling of blood products, and the use of antibiotics have greatly improved the safety of cesarean section. Further, one criticism of elective cesareans in the past was that they were inadvertently performed too early, before the baby's lungs were mature enough. This miscalculation is preventable today with ultrasound and more precise techniques of dating the age of the fetus than simply projecting from the date of the last menstrual period.

One thing that physicians continue to discuss and dispute is the selection of women who are good candidates for VBAC. The question of safety is trickier if you have had more than one cesarean, if your current baby is breech, if you are carrying twins, or if you have a low vertical scar or an unknown uterine scar (again, your uterine scar may be different from the external scar on your skin).

For instance, if your current baby is breech, the majority of doctors would still say that it is unwise to subject your scarred uterus to the added stress of external version to try to turn the baby to a head-down position. However, a growing number of doctors are comfortable performing external version on women with a scarred uterus—if the uterus can tolerate labor, they argue, it can handle a gentle attempt to move the baby—as long as it is late enough in the pregnancy for the baby to be delivered (37 weeks) if labor starts and it is done in a labor and delivery room.

Doctors also do not universally agree on what to do in a VBAC candidate whose baby remains breech. Some would allow a trial of labor, but most probably would not. Not many such women have been studied, and since breech presentation occurs in just 3 to 4 percent of all pregnancies, even high-profile, pro-VBAC doctors such as Bruce Flamm don't see this group as a good target for substantially lowering the cesarean section rate.

Besides arguing about who is and isn't a good candidate for VBAC, doctors also differ on how aggressively to recommend VBAC to their patients (the choice issue again) and, in women who do have a trial of labor, how aggressively to pursue it when the labor road gets bumpy.

Physicians who strongly favor a trial of labor argue that vaginal delivery is safer for the mother than elective cesarean because it avoids surgery. When you take a large group of attempted VBACs, including successes and failures, they say, the overall rate of complications to mothers is less than that for elective cesarean.

Conversely, other physicians contend that, while VBAC is a fine option for carefully selected, well-motivated candidates, elective cesarean may confer fewer risks to the baby. And when a trial of labor fails, they say, the risk of complications may be higher for both mother and baby.

How Risks Are Defined

In categorizing risks, physicians talk about maternal mortality, maternal morbidity, perinatal mortality, and perinatal morbidity. Maternal mortality means death of the mother associated directly with pregnancy or childbirth. Morbidity means complications. Maternal mortality rates in the United States have improved dramatically in the past fifty years, and today the rate is expressed in terms of deaths per 100,000 live births. In 1992, the maternal mortality rate was 7.8 (per 100,000 live births), according to the National Center for Health Statistics.

While there is no universal definition of what constitutes morbidity for the mother, most studies include hemorrhage, the need for a blood transfusion, the need for a hysterectomy, infection, fever, endometritis (inflammation of the uterine lining due to infection), extended hospital stay, and separation or rupture of the uterine scar; a few also include damage to the perineum (the tissue from the genitals to the anus).

When discussing babies, doctors differentiate between the terms *fetal*, *neonatal*, and *perinatal*. Fetal is typically the term used before birth. A fetal death means the baby died in utero and was stillborn. A neonate is a newborn. An early neonatal death is one that occurs in the first seven days of life, while a late neonatal death occurs after seven days but before twenty-eight days. The perinatal mortality rate (PMR) is the sum of fetal and neonatal deaths and is expressed in terms of deaths per 1000 total births (including stillbirths). When statisticians speak of infants, they are referring to babies under one year of age.

Statistically, childbirth is far more dangerous to the baby than to the mother. According to *Williams Obstetrics*, there are currently 180 perinatal deaths for every maternal death. "With the current very low incidence of maternal deaths, perinatal loss rates not only are a better index of the level of obstetrical care, but also give a valid indication of an equally important obstetrical indicator, *infant morbidity*," write the authors. Fortunately, perinatal mortality rates have fallen dramatically in the past forty years, from 39.0 per 1000 in 1950 to 12.8 in 1992, according to Ken Schoendorf, M.D., MPH, a medical epidemiologist at the National Center for Health Statistics.

Infant morbidity includes low birthweight and congenital abnormalities. Since neither of these problems is related to the method of delivery, they aren't relevant to a discussion of the merits of VBAC versus repeat cesarean. In most medical papers on VBAC, infant morbidity is defined as the need for intensive care, external injuries such as fractures or large bruises, seizures, and, most frequently, low 1-minute and 5-minute Apgar scores. Many doctors now believe that a test of the baby's blood taken immediately after delivery, called "umbilical cord arterial blood pH," is a better indicator of the baby's condition and long-term health prognosis than Apgar scores. (Apgar scores may also be falsely low in premature infants who are otherwise healthy.) But nearly all the studies to date comparing VBAC to elective repeat cesarean have used Apgar scores as the indicator of the baby's condition, without including umbilical cord blood pH.

Apgar scores are taken at 1 minute and 5 minutes after birth. The baby receives a score of 0, 1, or 2 points in each of five categories: heart rate (0 if absent, 1 if below 100, 2 if over 100); respiratory rate (0 if absent, 1 if slow and irregular, 2 if good, crying); reflex response (0 if no response, 1 if grimace, 2 if vigorous cry); muscle tone (0 if flaccid, 1 if some flexion of extremities, 2 if active motion); and color (0 if blue or pale, 1 if body is pink but extremities blue, 2 if completely pink).

Table 5 Apgar Scores			
What Is evaluated	Score of 0	Score of 1	Score of 2
Heart rate	Absent	Less than 100	More than 100
Respiration	Absent	Slow and irregular	Good, crying
Reflex response	No response	Grimace	Vigorous cry
Muscle tone	Limp	Moves extremities	Is active
Color	Blue, pale	Body pink, extremities blue	All pink

Note: Apgar scores are taken 1 minute after birth and again at 5 minutes after birth. A low 1-minute score (0 to 3) means immediate intervention is necessary to resuscitate the baby. A 1-minute score of 4 to 6 may mean the baby is moderately depressed. A score of 7 to 10 means the baby is in excellent condition. In physiologically mature, normal infants, the 5-minute score should be between 7 and 10. This method was devised by Dr. Virginia Apgar in 1952.

The 1-minute score is not a good predictor of the baby's future health but is useful in determining whether the baby needs immediate medical attention, namely resuscitation. A 1-minute score of 7 to 10 means the baby is in excellent condition; a score of 4 to 6 means the baby is moderately depressed, with slow breathing but good heart rate; and a score of 0 to 3 means the baby is severely depressed and needs to be resuscitated.

A normal 5-minute score is between 7 and 10. Scores between 4 and 6 constitute a gray area, but more likely than not the baby will be fine. A score of 0 to 3 is associated with a slightly increased risk of cerebral palsy. However, according to *Williams Obstetrics*, a baby with a 5-minute score of 0 to 3 that improves to 4 or better at 10 minutes has a 99 percent chance of not having cerebral palsy at age 7.

Unfortunately, when an apparently healthy child develops a learning disorder or behavioral or health problem at a later age, there is no good way of determining whether the birth experience may have contributed to the cause.

Risks to the Mother

Most physicians and statisticians would agree that cesarean delivery is associated with greater risks for the mother than vaginal delivery.

Cesarean delivery

The risks of cesarean delivery are the same as for any major surgery. They include: infection; problems with general anesthesia, particularly the danger of choking on the stomach contents (regional anesthesia eliminates this risk); excessive blood loss; and a small risk of pulmonary embolism, which can occur when a blood clot develops and travels to the lungs. Specific to cesarean surgery, a mistake can incur an injury to the bladder or nearby vessels. Some of the morbidity associated with the surgery, however, is related to the problem that led to the cesarean (such as placenta previa). In these cases, the risk of morbidity or mortality might have been greater with a vaginal delivery.

Interestingly, the Centers for Disease Control and Prevention, which includes the National Center for Health Statistics, has no statistics that can clearly distinguish maternal deaths related to cesarean from those related to vaginal delivery. The reason, says Hani Atrash, M.D., chief of the pregnancy and infant health branch at the CDC, is that in about 35 percent of all maternal deaths related to childbirth from 1979 to 1990, the method of delivery was not indicated on the birth certificate. So it's impossible in these cases to correlate the cause of death with the method of birth, and thus impossible to publish reliable national statistics.

"We are very careful about making statements about mortality following cesarean section," says Dr. Atrash. "I'm not promoting cesarean sections; I'm sure many more are performed than necessary, everybody agrees with that. But if you ask how many women and babies are we saving by doing c-sections, the outcome would be we are saving many more than we are losing. Complications following cesarean may be higher than complications following vaginal delivery. However, we need to keep in mind that many of those women who were sectioned would have had serious complications or died, and many of those babies would have died if they were not sectioned." A national goal of a 12 to 15 percent cesarean rate is logical, he says. By contrast, in countries such as Brazil, where the cesarean rate is as high as 90 percent in some hospitals, the risks are clearly outweighing the benefits. On the other hand, in developing countries with a 5 percent cesarean rate, women who need cesareans aren't getting them.

Of further note, a study cited in *Williams Obstetrics* found that in the state of Massachusetts between 1976 and 1984, only 7 deaths following more than 121,000 cesareans could be directly attributed to the surgery (a rate of 5.8 per 100,000). Another study published in 1990 found that the risk of maternal death was five times greater for cesarean than vaginal delivery, after complications of the pregnancy itself were excluded. The same study found that the risk of dying in an emergency cesarean was 1.4 times greater than in an elective cesarean.

Since any major surgery poses certain risks, including cesarean, it's especially important for doctors not to treat it trivially and not to perform a first cesarean without just cause. However, even for the patient who ends up with an emergency operation to save a life, the odds of something terrible happening are very low. The risks of elective cesarean are lower still, which makes the choice a difficult one for the VBAC candidate, who also has to evaluate the risks of labor following cesarean as well as the risks of ending up with an emergency cesarean.

Trial of labor versus elective repeat cesarean

While few studies have actually compared maternal outcomes for elective repeat cesarean and trial of labor, many have examined trial of labor in isolation. In a study published in 1990, VBAC researcher Bruce Flamm analyzed 5,733 trials of labor in eight California Kaiser Permanente hospitals over a five-year period from 1984 to 1989. The VBAC rate was 75 percent, and there were no maternal deaths. There were just ten cases of uterine rupture (0.17 percent), leading to two hysterectomies. Dr. Flamm's conclusion: the policy of routine repeat cesarean should be replaced by a trial of labor in selected candidates.

One criticism voiced by the more cautious contingent of doctors is that there still has not been a randomized, controlled study comparing maternal and neonatal outcomes between trial of labor and elective repeat cesarean. Such a study would *randomly* assign a large group of VBAC-eligible mothers to either a trial of labor or an elective cesarean and then look at the outcomes. The next best thing is to compare outcomes between the two groups even though they are not randomly assigned but self-selected. In a telephone interview, I asked Dr. Flamm why his initial study didn't include a control group of women who opted for repeat cesarean.

"The decision was never to see if this is better or safer than elective repeat cesarean," he said. "The goal was just to say, is it a reasonable thing to do?" In a more recent paper (1994), Dr. Flamm did compare the two groups, consisting of 7,229 women who delivered at ten Southern California Kaiser Permanente hospitals. Of these, 5,022 had a trial of labor, with 3,746 (75 percent) succeeding and 1,276 ending up with a repeat cesarean. (Women were excluded from a trial of labor if they had a low vertical or classical vertical scar, but not if their scar type was undocumented in their chart.) The remaining 2,207 women elected to have a repeat cesarean. The study does not distinguish outcomes between women who succeeded and failed at VBAC but compares the entire trial-of-labor group with the elective-cesarean group.

Here are the statistically significant differences. The hospital stay averaged 27 hours less for the trial-of-labor group than the elective-cesarean group. The trial-of-labor group had lower rates of transfusion (0.72 percent versus 1.72 percent) and lower rates of postpartum fever (12.7 percent versus 16.4 percent). There were 39 uterine ruptures in the trial-of-labor group (0.78 percent), resulting in three hysterectomies.

Combined with Dr. Flamm's previous VBAC studies, this paper brings the number of trials of labor studied at the Southern California Kaiser hospitals to more than 10,000. There was a single maternal death in a trial-of-labor candidate who died when an emergency cesarean section had to be performed due to fetal distress. She was put under general anesthesia and died of complications from aspirating her stomach contents. (Is it fair to suggest that she probably would have survived an elective repeat cesarean under epidural anesthesia?)

Hysterectomy for a rupture that could not be repaired occurred in less than 1 per 2000 labors. (The rate of rupture increased from 0.2 percent in his earlier studies to 0.8 percent in the current study.)

"From all the data we looked at, trial of labor looked better than elective repeat cesarean," Dr. Flamm says. "Now certainly it's not big differences, and it's not showing that elective repeat cesarean is a horrendous thing. What I'm arguing more is just if someone doesn't need major surgery, we probably shouldn't do it.

"A trial of labor doesn't have to be fifteen hours long," he adds. "Some people have misconceptions about that, but I think it's worth giving it a chance. If things are going great and the baby's heart rate looks good on the monitor and the cervix is dilating quickly, in many cases you can have a nice, normal birth and avoid a cesarean. That doesn't mean that every woman has to have some kind of acid test."

A small study of 75 women with one low transverse cesarean section who were offered a trial of labor was conducted at the Hospital of the University of Pennsylvania in Philadelphia by Carolyn Hadley, M.D. Forty of the 75 women had a trial of labor, with 32 delivering vaginally (80 percent) and 8 having a repeat cesarean. The other 35 had an elective repeat cesarean.

There were no uterine ruptures and no emergency hysterectomies. The percentage of women with complications such as fever, endometritis, and other infections was nearly identical in the cesarean group (25.6 percent) and the trial-of-labor group overall (25.0 percent). But 50 percent of the women whose trial of labor ended in repeat cesarean had such complications, as compared to 15.6 percent of the women whose trial of labor succeeded. The authors conclude that their findings do not favor one method of delivery over the other.

A number of other studies have also found that women with successful VBACs have lower rates of complications than women with repeat cesareans, but that women with failed trials of labor have complications at a comparable rate to women having a primary non-elective cesarean after failure to progress in labor.

A 1991 paper by Dr. Mortimer Rosen at Presbyterian Hospital in New York City looked at thirty-one studies with a total of 11,417 trials of labor. There were two maternal deaths in the study population, one due to a fatal pulmonary embolism after a failed trial of labor and one involving a repeat cesarean for a woman at 32 weeks' gestation with placenta accreta (implantation of the placenta into the uterine wall, which can cause infection and hemorrhage).

The risk of uterine rupture or scar dehiscence (see "Uterine rupture" below) for a failed trial of labor was 2.8 times greater than for elective repeat cesarean. The rate of complications related to fever (called *febrile morbidity*, which includes various kinds of infections) was twice as high in the failed-trial-of-labor group as in the elective-cesarean group but only one fifth as high in the successful VBAC group as in the elective-cesarean group.

Uterine rupture

Though the incidence of uterine rupture in women with a low transverse incision from one previous cesarean is less than 1 percent, every such woman is at risk because there is no way of telling ahead of time which uterus will rupture. The fact that the risk is relatively low could lead to complacency and lack of attentiveness on the part of the attendants managing your labor. Uterine ruptures can be repaired without hysterectomy and without ill effects to the baby, but they must be diagnosed and treated immediately to avoid more catastrophic consequences.

Study after study shows that the only consistent and reliable sign of uterine rupture is a sudden and lasting deceleration of the baby's heart rate, without prior warning and often without symptoms felt by the mother. The only method for continuous monitoring of the baby's heart rate is electronic fetal monitoring. If you plan to have a trial of labor, you owe it to yourself to make absolutely sure ahead of time that your labor will be electronically monitored at all times, that someone skilled in reading monitors is either always in your room or close by, and that your hospital's staff has the skill and the resources to respond quickly in the event of such an emergency.

Many papers have been written about uterine rupture, and the findings tend to be similar. One expert who has reported on uterine rupture is James R. Scott, M.D., chairman of the department of obstetrics and gynecology at the University of Utah Medical Center in Salt Lake City. It is important to distinguish between true uterine rupture and scar dehiscence, because one is dangerous while the other is so symptomless it may go undetected. In Dr. Scott's work, *uterine rupture* is defined as "complete separation of the wall of the pregnant uterus, with or without expulsion of the fetus, endangering the life of the mother or fetus." Typically there is fetal distress and acute maternal bleeding. *Scar dehiscence* is a small break or window in the scar that does not cause problems to mother or baby and that may only be detected by manually examining the uterus after delivery, a procedure that is itself somewhat controversial.

In a 1991 paper, Dr. Scott analyzed twelve uterine ruptures in the Salt Lake City area, ten of which occurred between 1987 and 1989. An addendum at the end of the paper reveals that two more ruptures occurred after the manuscript had been submitted but before it was published. Here is a summary paragraph about the consequences of the twelve ruptures:

> The range of estimated blood loss was 1–4 liters; transfusion was necessary in four cases and hysterectomy was required in two. All mothers survived, but six infants were severely depressed at birth, three perinatal deaths occurred, and two infants suffered neurologic impairment. In four cases with poor perinatal outcome, litigation has occurred or is in progress.

In the two ruptures that occurred after the manuscript was submitted, one mother gave birth to a moderately depressed infant who "has done well" and the uterus was repaired; in the other case, the uterus was also repaired and though emergency cesarean delivery was performed within 30 minutes after fetal distress was detected on the monitor, the baby was completely "extruded" through the scar (expelled from the uterus into the abdominal cavity) and did not survive.

Dr. Scott writes that eleven of the twelve women had previous low transverse incisions, while one had a low vertical incision. Of the eleven, he writes, ten would have been classified by most physicians as being at low risk for uterine rupture. The three fetal deaths all occurred "when the women were not under the direct observation of a physician with continuous fetal monitoring."

The rate of uterine rupture may be underreported, Dr. Scott writes, because of the "tendency to publish favorable but not unfavorable results." At his own hospital, for instance, a teaching hospital, the rate of uterine rupture in 196 trials of labor between 1982 and 1989 was 1.5 percent, higher than the rate published by most studies.

Dr. Scott expresses concern about several related issues. One is that smaller community hospitals where many women give birth may not have the staff or equipment to respond quickly enough to the emergency presented by a ruptured uterus.

"I'm not sure everybody in the ivory towers understands what docs and patients can do in smaller community hospitals," Dr. Scott said in a telephone interview. "The recommendation is that you should be able to do a cesarean section within 15 to 30 minutes for a uterine rupture, and that there should be in-house obstetric and in-house anesthesia coverage. If you are out in some rural area, there just isn't 24-hour in-house coverage. I was in general practice in rural Iowa before I went into ob-gyn, and I would not be anxious to do VBACs in that particular situation, because we really couldn't have handled it if somebody had a ruptured uterus. We just wouldn't get people there fast enough."

Second, he wonders if the criteria for promoting a trial of labor are getting too lax. "Although patients were selected carefully in the initial studies," he writes, "there is now an expanding list of obstetric conditions reportedly appropriate for vaginal birth after cesarean. Usually studied in small series, these conditions include multiple previous cesareans, unknown uterine scars, breech presentation, twins, post-term pregnancy, and suspected macrosomia."

Dr. Scott is not against VBAC. "I'm supportive of VBAC, and I think it's a reasonable procedure," he says. "But the thing we have to be careful about is that as VBAC becomes more and more accepted, it's becoming more and more casual. There is approximately a 1 percent risk of uterine rupture in VBACs, and that's not high but it's not insignificant. So I don't think it's something that should be done casually."

Uterine rupture and arrest disorders

While all women with a low transverse incision are at risk for uterine rupture, events during labor may further predispose a woman to that danger. A group of researchers, led by Anna S. Leung, M.D., at the University of Southern California in Los Angeles compared a group of 70 women who suffered a uterine rupture during a trial of labor after a previous cesarean with a randomly selected group of 70 women who did not (the control group). The study found that three variables were associated with an increased risk of uterine rupture:

- Excessive use of Pitocin. "Our study confirmed that over-use of oxytocin was associated with increased risk of uterine rupture," they write. The authors define overuse as the administration of Pitocin to make the cervix dilate faster in the latent (early) phase of labor, even when there are no signs of dysfunction. The authors attribute the excessive use to the fact that the resident physicians in the study were "constantly caring for a large number of patients and could not await labor progress." In other words, they were rushed. The authors recommend the alternative course of therapeutic rest, which consists of giving the mother a narcotic and letting her relax until labor progresses on its own, though they concede this method takes longer.

- Dysfunctional labor itself. Only 10 percent of the control group had dysfunctional labor, compared to 44 percent of the case group. The study's authors calculated that women with dysfunctional labor had a rate of rupture 7.2 times greater than that of women with normal labor. Labor was considered dysfunctional if the latent phase lasted longer than fourteen hours; if dilation occurred at a rate less than 1.5 centimeters per hour during the active phase; if dilation stopped during the active phase for two hours or more (arrest of dilation); or if the descent of the baby's presenting part stopped for an hour or more (arrest of descent).

- Women with a history of two or more cesareans had a rate of rupture 2.6 times greater than that of women with just one cesarean.

The features that were not associated with uterine rupture in the study are equally interesting. They include epidural anesthesia, a birthweight greater than 4000 grams (8 lbs. 13 oz.), and a history of cesarean section for cephalopelvic disproportion. A history of successful vaginal delivery after cesarean section didn't raise or lower the risk of uterine rupture.

In addition to warning against the overzealous use of Pitocin in early labor, the authors recommend that cesarean section should be considered promptly if attempts to resolve arrest disorders with the judicious use of Pitocin have no effect. (It is not overly difficult to tell whether the Pitocin is not working: though the Pitocin cranks up the contractions to an adequate strength, as determined by an intrauterine pressure catheter, the cervix still doesn't dilate further. This is why cesareans are performed for "arrest of labor" or "failure to progress.") In general, women who experience arrest disorders have a lower prognosis for vaginal delivery.

If you experienced an arrest disorder that lasted two hours or longer in a previous pregnancy, you may want to discuss alternative plans in advance of delivery with your doctor in the event it happens again. A 1994 study of 2,709 vaginal and 764 cesarean deliveries by M. Maurice Abitbol, M.D., at University Hospital in Stony Brook, New York, found that the longer the arrest of labor, the greater the maternal morbidity, regardless of the type of delivery. Morbidity included excessive tearing of either cesarean scars or vaginal or cervical tissue that required suturing (and which occurred in spite of episiotomies), hemorrhage, fever, urinary retention, wound complications, and extended length of stay.

While the rate of complications was higher for cesarean delivery than vaginal delivery overall, the lowest rate of complications (1.9 and 2.0 percent) occurred in women with vaginal and elective cesarean deliveries who had no arrest of labor.

In women with arrest of labor lasting two to three hours, those who delivered vaginally had a 33 percent rate of complications compared to 6.9 percent for the cesarean group. When arrest lasted three to five hours (all of these women ended up with cesareans), the rate of complications rose to 29 percent. Among patients whose arrest was allowed to continue for more than five hours (also all cesareans), the rate of complications was 100 percent.

In 67 cases of prolonged arrest (more than two hours with no epidural or more than three hours with epidural) that occurred before the women were fully dilated, all required cesarean delivery. "We believe that if a cesarean delivery had been performed in these 67 cases before the arrest became prolonged, the numerous maternal complications may have been avoided," writes Dr. Abitbol. "This approach would not increase the cesarean delivery rate."

Lacerations

Vaginal delivery in general carries risk of damage to the perineal area (the external area from the vagina to the anus) as well as to the cervix and the rectum. In women attempting VBAC, the rate of such complications may be greater than in women who deliver their first or subsequent child vaginally.

Though few studies exist on this topic, one paper by Thomas Yetman, M.D. and Thomas E. Nolan, M.D., at the U.S. Naval Hospital in Portsmouth, Virginia, compared the perineal complications of a group of 224 women who attempted VBAC with a group of women who were attempting their first vaginal delivery as well as with a larger control group of women with vaginal deliveries, including those with one or more previous vaginal deliveries. The study defined a "significant laceration" as one designated on the delivery summary as third degree ("complete disruption of the rectal sphincter with intact rectal mucosa"; mucosa is the innermost lining), fourth degree ("disruption of the rectal mucosa and the sphincter muscle"), vault ("tears of the vaginal walls"), or cervical ("lacerations of the cervix that require repair").

Among the 137 women with successful VBACs, the rate of significant perineal lacerations was 35.8 percent, compared with 24.9 percent in the group having a first vaginal delivery and 17.9 percent in the vaginal delivery control group. The authors note that these differences occurred even though the VBAC women were cared for by more highly trained physicians than the others.

In addition, there was a higher risk of repeat cesarean for women whose babies weighed more than 3720 grams (8 lbs. 3 oz.), and those with babies weighing more than 3600 grams (7 lbs. 15 oz.) who did deliver vaginally had a higher rate of significant lacerations (49.0 percent versus 28.9 percent). "We believe

that gravidas [pregnant women] who consider a vaginal birth after cesarean section attempt should be counseled with regard to
the increased incidence of lacerations and that this possibility
(along with the resultant possibility of long-term sequelae such as
rectovaginal fistulae [an abnormal passage between the rectum
and the vagina]) should be part of the decision to undertake a
vaginal birth after cesarean section."

Significant lacerations tend to occur more frequently when forceps are used to achieve vaginal delivery. The use of forceps itself
varies widely depending on geographic region and from hospital
to hospital, as does the medical school training in their use. Some
doctors are well skilled in their use, while others aren't.

In the Portsmouth study, forceps were used in 10.2 percent of
the VBAC attempts, 9.5 percent in the first attempt at vaginal
delivery, and 5.0 percent in the women with one or more previous vaginal deliveries. Significant lacerations occurred in 56
percent of the VBAC group when forceps were used, 44 percent
of the first-vaginal-delivery group, and 49 percent in the mothers
with more vaginal deliveries. Though the differences between the
groups who had forceps was insignificant, the incidence of lacerations was much higher in all the forceps groups than in the
groups who delivered spontaneously.

For a time, forceps and vacuum extraction (a newer method of
pulling the baby down) seemed to fall out of favor because of
questions about their safety for mother and baby. However, there
appears to be a resurgence in their use, especially because forceps
can represent a final effort to deliver a baby vaginally before resorting to cesarean. Though it has not been widely documented,
doctors who push VBACs may tend to use forceps more frequently in VBAC patients. One paper by Paul Meier, M.D., and
Richard Porreco, M.D., reported a 23 percent incidence of forceps or vacuum extractor use in 175 successful VBACs. (They did
not report the corresponding incidence of lacerations.)

There appears to be an association between increased use of
epidural anesthesia and the use of forceps, according to *Williams
Obstetrics*. Epidurals can prompt the need for forceps if the ability
to push is impaired. During prenatal care, you may wish to dis-

cuss whether your doctor uses forceps or vacuum extraction, how frequently, and under what circumstances, and think about whether you would prefer to risk the added perineal trauma from forceps, which can be significant, or the possible surgical complications from a cesarean.

To summarize, medical risks to the mother who has surgery include a longer hospital stay, a higher incidence of fever, and the greater likelihood of needing a transfusion. Elective surgery has a lower rate of morbidity than emergency surgery. The risks of laboring after a cesarean include uterine rupture and perineal lacerations. Lacerations are more likely if forceps are used. The morbidity rates of elective cesarean and trial of labor are fairly similar.

For some women, the most resonant risk of laboring is the risk of ending up with another cesarean. For others, it's a matter of selecting one set of risks over the other. For instance, are you more worried about the possibility of needing a transfusion (you may be able to arrange to donate your own blood ahead of time, unless you are anemic) or the possibility of uterine rupture? Are you more concerned about spending two extra days in the hospital, in the event of surgery, or about the possibility of having perineal lacerations?

Risks to the Baby

A dictum in obstetrics holds that in rare and unfortunate situations in which the mother's and baby's health are both endangered, the mother's health always comes first. But more often than not, the baby is the one at greater risk in the labor and delivery room. The majority of obstetrical malpractice lawsuits fall into two categories: failure to perform a cesarean section and improper use of forceps. These are typically situations resulting in the death or severe damage of the baby, not the mother.

The findings that VBAC is slightly riskier for the baby than elective repeat cesarean are consistent and widespread, yet pro-VBAC authors tend to downplay their own findings. In a 1989 paper about the risk of VBAC in large babies, with regard to damage caused by difficulty in delivering the shoulders, Dr. Flamm writes that "it has been estimated that a policy of elective cesarean section for estimated fetal weight over 4500 grams would result in 978 cesarean operations for each case of mild persistent arm weakness prevented." Apparently, the vaginal delivery of the one infant with persistent arm weakness justifies the savings of 978 cesarean operations to Dr. Flamm. Statistically, this may be a sound premise in women who are capable of delivering very large babies vaginally, but what would you prefer: a repeat cesarean and a healthy baby, or a VBAC and a baby with persistent arm weakness?

Dr. Flamm and other VBAC advocates argue that Apgar scores, their own choice of measurement for infant well-being, are of questionable value in assessing long-term infant health, and yet they don't include other measures such as cord blood pH. Also, because of technological advances in neonatal emergency care, which are wonderful and lifesaving, some doctors treat these high-tech interventions fairly casually. If a baby with a low 1-minute Apgar score can be successfully resuscitated with techniques such as intubating and CPR, it matters less to the attending physician that the baby had the low score in the first place. But most mothers, presumably, would be happier with a pink baby that breathes on its own than a bluish, unconscious one that needs an immediate intervention.

In Dr. Flamm's five-year study of trial of labor with no control group (see page 62), one baby died as a result of uterine rupture and another developed signs of cerebral palsy. Though the corrected perinatal mortality rate was low (9 per 1000), one baby in distress died as a result of a vacuum-assisted delivery. Dr. Flamm writes that since there was no uterine rupture in the mother, the death was "felt to be totally unrelated to the previous cesarean scar." The death was clearly related to the VBAC however, and the baby would have been saved by elective repeat cesarean. Dr. Flamm and other pro-VBAC practitioners argue that such incidents cannot be blamed on VBAC because they could just as easily happen in any vaginal delivery. In other words, they seem to be saying, if something goes wrong in a VBAC that isn't related to the scar, you can't blame it on VBAC.

Cesarean delivery

In the past, the biggest risk of elective surgery to the baby was due to iatrogenic (doctor induced) prematurity. Babies delivered too early suffered from respiratory distress because their lungs were immature. However, newer methods for determining gestational age, such as ultrasound early in pregnancy, have largely eliminated this risk. According to *Williams Obstetrics*, the risk of respiratory distress is not significantly different in vaginally delivered babies and cesarean babies when the gestational ages are identical.

Other risks of cesarean include physical trauma to the baby, which may be caused by the incision or by the process of lifting the baby out. If a doctor does a transverse uterine incision in the case of a very small, preterm infant in breech position, there may be some difficulty getting the head out. This is why there's a need for vertical incisions in some cases. It's important to remember that there are also risks to preterm infants and breech infants in vaginal deliveries.

When the position and gestational age of the baby is known and the doctor is skilled, cesarean delivery is a very safe procedure for the baby. In the 1300-plus page text of *Williams Obstetrics*, only three short paragraphs are devoted to a discussion of perinatal mortality and morbidity from cesarean section. The paragraph on mortality states that the frequency of death is affected by the underlying reason for the cesarean and the baby's age, not by the surgery itself.

Trial of labor versus elective repeat cesarean

The 1994 paper by Dr. Flamm comparing perinatal outcomes of elective repeat cesarean with trial of labor found that the trial-of-labor group had a higher percentage of babies with 5-minute Apgar scores of less than 7. The percentage of low-scoring infants was relatively small for both groups, however, totaling 0.68 percent for the cesarean mothers and 1.48 percent for the trial-of-labor mothers. The paper did not compare the perinatal mortality rates of the two groups, stating instead that the overall perinatal mortality rate of 7 per 1000 live births in the study population was similar to the combined rate of 10 per 1000 at all the hospitals participating in the study.

The aforementioned studies by Dr. Hadley and Dr. Rosen also compared perinatal outcomes of elective repeat cesarean with trial of labor. In Hadley's groups, 3 of 35 babies delivered by elective cesarean required a total of 5 days' stay in a special-care nursery, while 4 of 40 babies in the trial-of-labor group (all in the successful VBAC group) required a total of 8 days' stay in the nursery. Hadley concludes that her group's findings do not favor either method of delivery.

In Dr. Rosen's meta-analysis, the overall perinatal mortality rates were 18 per 1000 live births for trial of labor versus 10 per 1000 for elective repeat cesarean. When stillbirths were eliminated, these numbers fell to 9 and 7 per 1000 respectively. (Some stillbirths, however, can be prevented by intervening early enough, at 38 to 39 weeks, with a cesarean section if a potential problem is identified or suspected. In fact, these numbers show that 9 stillbirths occurred for every 1000 live births for the trial-of-labor group, as opposed to 3 per 1000 for the cesarean group.) When stillbirths, very low birthweight babies, and congenital abnormalities were excluded from the data, the mortality rates dropped to 3 per 1000 for trial of labor and 4 per 1000 for elective repeat cesarean. Based on these findings, there is no significant difference in perinatal mortality rates between trial of labor and elective repeat cesarean.

In terms of morbidity for the babies, those born after a trial of labor had low 5-minute Apgar scores 2.1 times as often as did the cesarean babies, but the data were not detailed enough to exclude low birthweight babies or those with serious congenital problems (which tend to be born vaginally, according to the authors). Nevertheless, while the chance of receiving a low 5-minute Apgar score was similar for the successful-VBAC group and the elective-cesarean group, the chance of having a low-scoring baby was 2.6 times greater after a failed trial of labor than after elective repeat cesarean.

One of the largest studies of the effects on babies of vaginal birth after cesarean was conducted at University College in Galway, Ireland. In a 1989 paper published in the *American Journal of*

Perinatology, Fergus P. Meehan and others reported on the perinatal outcomes in 1,498 women with one or more prior cesareans who delivered a total of 1,518 babies between 1972 and 1982 (the 20 extra babies were delivered to 18 mothers with twins and one with triplets). Of the 1,498 women, 654 had elective repeat cesarean (all had had two or more prior cesareans) and 844 had a trial of labor. Of the 844, 702 (83 percent) delivered vaginally, and 142 ended up with repeat operations.

The results of the study are grim by American standards. There were 46 perinatal deaths among the 1518 babies, for an overall perinatal mortality rate (PMR) of 30.3 (meaning 30.3 deaths out of 1000). Four of the babies died as a direct result of uterine rupture.

Starting with the best results, there were 7 deaths among 662 babies delivered by elective repeat cesarean, for a PMR of 10.6; 26 deaths among 712 babies delivered vaginally for a PMR of *36.5*; and 13 deaths among 144 babies delivered by emergency repeat cesarean for a PMR of *90.3*. When babies with congenital abnormalities were subtracted, the corrected PMRs were *4.5* for elective cesarean section and *29.2* for trial of labor.

To put these numbers into perspective, the hospital's overall PMR for the entire study period, during which more than 27,000 babies were delivered, was 22.5. The authors also state that the PMR for trial-of-labor patients decreased over the ten-year period from 40 to 20. They attribute this improvement to wider use of ultrasound during pregnancy, the increase from almost no electronic fetal monitoring during labor in the early years of the study to its routine use by the end of the study, and the existence in later years of a more sophisticated neonatal intensive care unit.

Still, as the authors point out, the corrected infant death rate associated with trial of labor was *six times* the rate associated with elective repeat cesarean. The hospital's policy regarding elective repeat cesarean is to perform the operation between 38 and 39 weeks' gestation, which is common in the United States as well. With regard to babies who were stillborn, the authors comment, "We believe . . . that four, and possibly six, babies might not have died had elective RCS been used at 38 weeks."

In contrast to most American studies, which assert that a trial of labor after previous cesarean section is safe, the authors of the Irish study take a much more cautious approach. "Attempted vaginal delivery after previous cesarean section is clearly a high-risk situation for both mother and fetus, and extreme vigilance is required of the attendant medical staff," they write. "Emphasis has in the past been laid on the possibility of uterine rupture with the resulting danger to mother and fetus. Although we advocate vaginal delivery after cesarean section, we believe the increased risk to the fetus in the procedure per se, as reported herein, has not been stressed sufficiently."

These findings underscore the importance of careful electronic monitoring in VBAC trials as well as the need for immediate access to neonatal intensive care facilities whenever trial of labor is attempted.

Uterine rupture

As the aforementioned paper by Dr. Scott at the University of Utah demonstrates, uterine rupture can be catastrophic to babies and mothers alike. Among the twelve uterine ruptures reported by Dr. Scott, plus the two later ruptures, a total of four babies died.

Though this may be difficult for the faint of heart to read, the babies who died were usually "extruded into the abdomen" of the mother. Because of the high pressure in the uterus during labor, when a rupture occurs, the tendency is for the baby and sometimes the placenta and umbilical cord to migrate to the opening in the uterine wall. When the mother's blood supply to the placenta suddenly drops as a result of hemorrhage or shock, the baby's oxygen supply can become compromised, resulting in fetal distress. This is why it is so crucial to have a medical team on hand that can rapidly deliver the baby and repair the mother's uterus.

Of the remaining ten babies, two were severely damaged with "residual neurologic sequelae," and the remaining eight, all with good 5-minute Apgar scores, were healthy infants.

What exactly does "severe residual neurologic sequelae" mean? In one case, a boy, born in 1986, is paralyzed as a result of oxygen deprivation to the brain and is never expected to walk, talk, or be able to take care of himself. The parents sued their doctor and their HMO, contending that the doctor should have planned an elective cesarean section instead of a trial of labor. The mother had a low vertical uterine incision with a breech infant in her first pregnancy. In addition, she had an abnormality called a *bicornuate uterus* (a uterus divided into two separate parts), such that the incision was done on one side of the uterus. No research exists to support the safety of a trial of labor in such cases.

The family's attorney claimed that the HMO's cost-cutting measures, such as giving doctors bonuses for keeping their expenses down (an incentive favoring VBAC over repeat cesarean), were partly to blame. But the jury assigned 100 percent of the fault to the doctor—90 percent for planning the VBAC and 10 percent for not warning the mother of the risks. The jury awarded the family $8.1 million.

Finally, in the study by Drs. Yetman and Nolan, (see page 70) there were four babies, among 224 attempted vaginal deliveries, with 5-minute Apgar scores of 6 or less. Two of these babies died, for a PMR of 8.93. One was a normal baby found to have died in utero at 41 weeks' gestation, presumably from a cord accident, according to the authors, in a woman planning a trial of labor. The other baby succumbed to a severe infection in the neonatal intensive care unit after the mother's trial of labor (post–42 weeks' gestation) ended in a repeat cesarean due to fetal distress.

"It is sobering to note that although neither of these deaths could be directly attributed to the vaginal birth after cesarean attempt, both of these infants probably would have survived the perinatal period had the mothers elected a repeat cesarean delivery rather than a vaginal birth after cesarean section," comment the authors.

Hindsight is always twenty-twenty, however, and as the expectant mother, you need to evaluate your history, your body, your psyche, and even what you can about your baby, such as his size, ahead of time. Serious complications to the infant due to a trial of labor are relatively rare, but they can occur. If you and your doctor are committed to a trial of labor, the most important things to remember, besides the need for high-level care and vigilance, are to remain flexible and not to be too overzealous in the goal to deliver vaginally, in the event an emergency arises.

While this chapter has included more of the negative possibilities than most doctors would ever volunteer to tell you, the fact remains that both elective repeat cesarean and an attempted VBAC, in well-selected women, are safe procedures when the health care professionals and the hospital staff are on their toes. As Dr. Leslie Iffy of New Jersey Medical School says, "So often in medicine, it's not so much a matter of what is being done, as how it is being done. I don't have a problem with a very carefully conducted attempt at VBAC, but I have a problem when people try to force it through and when physicians are overpersuaded that this is an innocent procedure. It is not."

FIVE

Why Half ·of Mothers Prefer Cesarean

If you are undecided about VBAC or flat out don't want it, you are not alone. Physicians striving to lower the cesarean rate by increasing their VBAC rate seem befuddled by this sizable group, about 40 to 50 percent of all women given the medical green light to pursue a VBAC. These physicians look at the medical and obstetric factors and say, "If the risks of VBAC and elective repeat cesarean are comparable, why choose surgery?"

More than befuddled, some physicians are downright annoyed by women who opt for surgery. "This latest ACOG guideline endorses a concept of management that obligates the obstetrician to include the patient in planning the approach to delivery," complains Gerald F. Joseph, Jr., M.D., lead author of a Louisiana study about patients who resisted a VBAC trial. Obviously, paternalistic physicians would rather not include the patient: they know what's best for you, your input doesn't count, and by golly, they are going to manage your labor and delivery the way they see fit. Unless, of course, you speak up and don't let them. The better informed you are about your options, the more they will be forced to take your demands seriously.

Unfortunately, sentiments ignoring the patient's wishes are quite common in the medical community. While focusing on the obstetric and economic factors that occupy physicians, the medical studies have a tendency to sweep over the psychological and social factors that affect your decision about the kind of childbirth you would prefer. Indeed, many studies are written as if the patient and her complex feelings about birth didn't exist. If the medical factors overwhelmingly favored one method over the other, this attitude would be more understandable. But when the medical risks of VBAC and repeat cesarean are fairly evenly balanced, there's no good reason for a doctor to insist on one method over the other.

Physicians Under Pressure

Like all of us, doctors are subject to pressures, even mandates, from peers and supervisors, including the very real and primarily economic pressure to lower the cesarean rate. Naturally, since elective repeat cesareans account for the biggest chunk of cesareans, VBAC candidates become good fodder for physicians striving to lower their own cesarean rate.

Let's say we have a qualified and talented obstetrician whose goal is to practice the best medicine possible. That physician looks at each pregnant patient neutrally, individually, and objectively. He (or she) treats each woman to the best of his ability, and if her pregnancy is uncomplicated, he hopes she will deliver vaginally but realizes circumstances may arise that could require a cesarean.

But now the physician must consider the mandate to lower the cesarean rate. Now he has an agenda to follow. How can he help but see every VBAC candidate as someone to chalk up on the VBAC scoreboard? Might not the pressure of this mandate color his ability to treat each patient neutrally and to practice the best medicine he possibly can? It's no wonder that the woman's preference becomes an annoyance, especially when it conflicts with his.

Let's assume the medical and obstetric risks of VBAC and cesarean section are comparable and that you are the VBAC candidate. Who should decide whether you have a trial of labor or an elective repeat cesarean—you, the physician, you and your physician together, or the insurance company?

If you are adamantly opposed to attempting a VBAC, should the physician keep pressuring you to try it anyway? What if the physician succeeds in persuading you, and then the trial of labor fails, and you end up with a repeat cesarean? Your baby is okay, but you are angry and disappointed with the experience, and you wish you had stuck to your instincts and had a cesarean in the first place. As long as you and the baby are okay, your physician is most likely satisfied. He may not take responsibility for disappointing you if he did what he thought was the right thing by convincing you to have a trial of labor. If you attempt a VBAC, you, not the physician, will have to cope with the emotional consequences if it doesn't work. If you opt for a repeat cesarean, there's less uncertainty about how you will feel, because you know what to expect.

Part Two of this book explores what other women in your predicament have done and how they felt. The rest of this chapter looks at several points of view in the medical journals about women's preferences and explanations for them.

Why Some Women Say No to VBAC

A study conducted by M. Maurice Abitbol, M.D. and others at Jamaica Hospital in New York examined why some women chose VBAC, why some chose repeat cesarean, and how everyone felt when it was over. The hospital followed 364 women with a cesarean in the previous pregnancy. Of these, 312 were considered good VBAC candidates—38 were excluded because of ACOG contraindications (previous scar unknown; fetal weight estimated at greater than 4000 grams, which is no longer an ACOG contraindication; baby wasn't in a head-down position; mother had gestational diabetes; or other reasons), and 14 more were excluded for reasons such as placenta previa, a prolapsed cord, or fetal death.

A social worker at the hospital held an initial meeting with the 312 VBAC candidates in which they were provided with the ACOG guidelines and told that their possibility of vaginal delivery was 50 to 80 percent. They were told that VBAC is associated with lower mortality rates for mothers and babies, that the hospital stay would be shorter and complications fewer, and that the circumstances leading to their previous cesarean would not necessarily recur. They also were informed of the possibility of uterine rupture and its consequences.

Each woman then had a private meeting with her physician and a social worker in which she was asked a set of standardized questions about her choice and her understanding of the potential complications of each procedure. If she expressed fear of pain during labor, she was reassured that adequate pain relief would always be available.

A third session was held for the women who had either decided against VBAC or couldn't make up their mind, but the study's authors say that while a VBAC trial was recommended for all 312 patients, at no time were the patients pressured to choose VBAC.

After they had delivered and before leaving the hospital, all 312 women were interviewed again about their feelings toward the outcome of their pregnancy.

Of the 312 eligible women, 125 (40 percent) opted for a repeat cesarean. Most of the women gave more than one reason, but the reason cited most often, by 71 percent of the women, "related to the negative emotional experience associated with the previous delivery—namely, prolonged and painful labor." This bears out what other studies have shown; that exceptionally long or difficult labors can leave psychological scars that are easily reopened. The women's responses also suggest that the physicians in their cesarean deliveries probably waited as long as they safely could for labor to progress before resorting to cesarean delivery. In other words, their cesareans were most likely not done for weak reasons.

Of the 187 women who opted to try VBAC, 65 (35 percent) ended up with a repeat cesarean. Of these 65 women, 49 "expressed varying degrees of frustration and even anger" about their experience, and those who had a long labor before being sectioned were "the most frustrated and disappointed." The other 16 women were also disappointed but said they would try VBAC again.

A substantial number of women experienced physical and emotional trauma from labor. It's easy for others with similar histories to empathize and to understand why these women wouldn't want to risk reliving such traumas. In fact, even more serious psychological consequences may occur when the same trauma strikes twice. But some obstetricians can't or refuse to relate to this.

"We get prepared psychologically for one thing and when it doesn't work out, it's extraordinarily traumatic, especially because we live in a culture where we actually believe we can control things by doing things right, going to Lamaze and doing all the right things," says Roneen Blank, M.D., describing the way some women feel after a cesarean. Dr. Blank is a psychiatrist and clinical director of the perinatal support services program at Good Samaritan Hospital in Downers Grove, Illinois.

"The next time there's the hope it can be different, it's a chance to rework the past," she says. "Part of what becomes so traumatizing is the repetition rather than the correction of the first event. And I don't think anyone prepares people for that."

Juxtapose her comments for a moment with the following. At Mount Sinai Hospital Medical Center in Chicago, a program was launched in 1985 to lower the hopital's cesarean rate. An article about the program, by Stephen A. Myers, M.D. and Norbert Cleicher, M.D., was published in the *New England Journal of Medicine* in 1988. The study, considered landmark by some who advocate stringent measures to lower the cesarean rate, told women at the hospital, who were primarily of a low socioeconomic background, that they would be expected to have a trial of labor after a previous cesarean. This included women with classical vertical scars and unknown scars and women who had undergone more than one cesarean.

"A patient's desire for a repeat cesarean section was not automatically accepted as an indication for that procedure," write the authors. "Only after prolonged consultation with the patient *and her family* were repeat cesareans performed at a patient's request" (emphasis added).

In addition, vaginal delivery was recommended for all babies who were breech, regardless of the type of breech, unless the head was hyperextended or fetal weight was estimated at more than 4300 grams (9 lbs. 8 oz.). The program succeeded in lowering the hospital's cesarean rate, from 17.5 percent to 11.5 percent, in two years. (Ironically, the decline in the repeat cesarean rate was not statistically significant.) But three of forty-eight breech babies died during vaginal delivery. That's a 6.25 percent infant mortality rate in this group, which is high. Moreover, the percentage of babies with 5-minute Apgar scores below 7 increased significantly, from 3.0 percent to 4.9 percent, during the study period. The authors suggest, not very convincingly, that this decline in infant health status was due to the "more stringent performance of Apgar assessments that began during the study period."

I do not believe that the end justified the means in this study. The women, who were primarily of low socioeconomic status, had all of their autonomy and choices in childbirth taken away from them. I wonder whether the risks of VBAC or of vaginal breech delivery were adequately explained to them, or explained at all. And because they were of low socioeconomic status, those whose babies were born with complications that might have been avoidable probably had no means of seeking recourse.

Unfortunately, paternalistic attitudes toward women in childbirth are still widespread. While many doctors will treat a woman with respect and take her choices seriously, others simply do not accept as valid a woman's reasons for wanting an elective repeat cesarean.

"Neither fear nor convenience constitutes justification for cesarean section," write Paul Meier, M.D, and Richard Porreco, M.D., in a 1982 study published in the *American Journal of Obstetrics and Gynecology*. "Rather, these factors identify areas which require further patient education and support." In his Denver practice today, Dr. Porreco does not grant patients a repeat cesarean that is not medically indicated, but he allows that he is happy to refer them to the practice next door. His position is that physicians need to exercise a choice with which they feel comfortable, just as patients do. He doesn't disagree with a woman's right to choose, but he won't treat her if the choice isn't in line with his. Unfortunately, because of growing constraints placed by insurance companies, not all women have the luxury of going to the doctor next door.

In the aforementioned New York study (see page 82), one group of women resisted VBAC but then accepted it "after extensive counseling," the nature of which was described as educational but not coercive. Of these 51 women, 33 succeeded and 18 had a repeat cesarean. Understandably, these last 18 were "most vocal in their complaints." But even more interestingly, 24 of the 33 who delivered vaginally were also dissatisfied with their experience. Maybe there's a lesson in this: if a woman really doesn't want a VBAC and especially if she isn't happy even when it works, who benefits by encouraging her to have one?

Childbirth is by nature unpredictable. Absolute happiness can't be guaranteed, and expectations about the process of labor and delivery are not always met. Some women might feel jubilant about a successful VBAC, while others won't. But a woman should at least be allowed to eliminate choices with which she is uncomfortable.

Fears associated with VBAC

Women in the New York study gave reasons other than negative emotional experience for refusing a VBAC. About 37 percent expressed concerns about the health of the baby. Such concerns, frequently dismissed by VBAC proponents, are not medically unfounded (see Chapter 4).

About 9 percent expressed fears that a difficult labor and delivery could "stretch the genital organs and tear the cervix, possibly resulting in problems such as uterine and vaginal prolapse, backache, difficult sexual intercourse and vaginal discharge." Since vaginal birth is considered the "natural and normal" way to deliver, damage incurred to the vagina, cervix, perineum, and anal region that may result from tearing, cutting, and pushing doesn't capture a great deal of attention from the traditionally male obstetrical community, though there are specialists, called *urogynecologists,* who try to fix such problems. These very real bodily afflictions are not usually counted in the "maternal morbidity" category (see Chapter 4).

Few, if any, studies exist that compare the effects of a cesarean with the effects of a vaginal birth on the quality of subsequent sexual intercourse. (Would the story be different if men were to routinely experience pain and difficulty with sexual intercourse or slow-healing wounds on their genital organs?) Isn't it understandable that a woman who has already had her abdominal wall cut would not feel very enthusiastic about having her vagina stretched and cut as well? Some women feel that one scar in one place is better than two scars in two places. (See Part Two for more direct reports from women about these problems.)

Convenience

Another controversial reason women in the New York study gave for wanting an elective repeat cesarean is the convenience factor. Many women would like to know and to help determine when the baby will arrive; the birth of a child, especially when there is already one or more at home, creates upheaval in a working family's life and often requires additional outside support, which may not be available at any time a woman happens to go into labor. Critics of this attitude ask, how dare women presume to want to have their babies when it's convenient for them? (Ironically, didn't cesareans that were scheduled for the convenience of physicians go unchallenged for a long time, until just recently?)

Unfortunately, the modern working world does not encourage the luxury of letting nature take its course any more. Most jobs permit a limited leave of absence, which many women can't afford to waste by taking time off before the delivery. Amidst all the organizing of the mother's schedule, the partner's schedule, the child's schedule, and the child's caretaker's schedule, a working woman facing a VBAC may have a nagging voice in the back of her mind asking whether this trial of labor is really going to work. Scheduling a delivery is one way of gaining a measure of control. In fact, some women and their doctors may schedule an induction instead of a repeat cesarean if the women don't go into labor by their due date or some designated point beyond. This can be an option, too.

Satisfaction with the birth experience

As mentioned above, the women who originally resisted a VBAC in the New York study but then accepted it had a high rate of dissatisfaction, regardless of the outcome. Looking at the women's satisfaction with the birth experience overall, 93 percent of the women who elected a repeat cesarean reported being satisfied, as opposed to 53 percent who opted for a VBAC trial. Among the 122 women whose VBAC succeeded, 68 percent were satisfied. In other words, one third were dissatisfied.

In the elective-cesarean group, only 7 percent of the women wished they had participated in the VBAC program or expressed interest in VBAC for a subsequent pregnancy.

Among the 122 women in the successful-VBAC group, 42 had complications. Complications included a prolonged active phase of labor (the middle phase, from about 4 to 7 centimeters), the use of forceps or vacuum extraction, temperature elevation in the mother, and excessive molding of the baby's head. The group without complications was 83 percent satisfied, while the group with complications was 55 percent dissatisfied.

Among the 65 women in the VBAC trial group who ended up with a repeat "indicated" (medically necessary) cesarean, 75 percent were dissatisfied. The reasons for cesarean section included arrest of labor during the active phase, progressive or sudden drops in the fetal heart rate, and temperature elevation in the mother.

The reasons for dissatisfaction are painfully apparent, as this group fared by far the worst in terms of outcome for mother and baby. One baby died as a result of uterine rupture in a mother with a previous low transverse incision, and the mother lost her uterus to an emergency hysterectomy. Four infants born to mothers in this group had 5-minute Apgar scores of less than 7, an indication of depressed breathing and circulatory functions. By comparison, among the babies born to the 125 elective-cesarean mothers, only one had a 5-minute Apgar of less than 7. Five mothers in the indicated cesarean group suffered complications, as opposed to none of the mothers in the elective-cesarean group. The authors state that nine of the indicated cesareans were difficult because the baby's head was stuck in the mother's midpelvic region. Eight of the indicated cesarean mothers required blood transfusions, as opposed to none in the elective group.

Among the 122 in the successful-VBAC group, four babies had 5-minute Apgar scores of less than 7, and two mothers had complications. One fetal death occurred, but it appears to have been unrelated to the mode of delivery.

Pro-choice doctors

The authors of the New York study state that their statistical conclusions do not differ greatly from other reports in the medical literature. In addition, an accompanying editorial in the journal, called "A Further View on the VBAC Quandary" by Maurice Abitbol, chairman of the department of obstetrics and gynecology at the Jamaica Hospital and lead author of the study, emphasizes that the hospital's true VBAC rate (the number of successful VBACs divided by the total number of women with previous cesareans, or 122/364) was 33.5 percent, which is comparable to the rate in other studies.

"My feeling is that as the proportion of patients having a VBAC trial goes above 50 percent," Dr. Abitbol writes, "the rate of failures and complications will also rise." He explains that it is misleading to tell the public that the success of VBAC is 60 to 80 percent because that figure applies only to the best candidates, women who are selected by their doctors and who also choose to try a VBAC. It is statistically inappropriate to extrapolate such figures to the population of cesarean mothers as a whole.

"My main point is we have to let women say what they want," he says. "I'm not saying one method is better than the other. I'm

just saying the freedom of choice has to be given to the patient."
For many women, he says, a trial of VBAC "increases the pain
and suffering of the patient and increases the risk of complications."

Why Women Choose VBAC

Another study conducted by Paul E. Kirk, M.D., and others in
Portland, Oregon, looked at the reasons for women's choices by
sending questionnaires to postpartum patients from University
Hospital, a public facility (A) and Good Samaritan Hospital, a
private hospital (B). A total of 111 patients, 70 from Hospital A
and 41 from Hospital B, planned a VBAC, and 77 percent succeeded. When asked to reveal the single most important factor
in their decision to choose VBAC, the answer that both groups
volunteered most often was the predicted longer recovery with
cesarean section, followed by the desire to experience vaginal
birth. The third most-often cited reason was "naturalness" of
vaginal birth (study's quotes). Though some women identified
"danger of cesarean section for mother" and "danger of cesarean
section for infant" on a given checklist of factors they considered in their decision, none of the 111 women who chose
VBAC identified either of these as the single most important
factor.

A total of 48 women, 15 from Hospital A and 33 from Hospital B, chose to have a repeat cesarean. The study's authors do not
say whether the women chose reasons from a list or whether they
could volunteer their own answers, but the women could cite
more than one reason for choosing cesarean section. The weight
they gave their reasons differed slightly between patients from the
two hospitals, but overall, 52 percent said they believed they had
a low probability of vaginal delivery. Other reasons, in order of
their overall importance to both groups combined, included
avoiding the pain of labor, knowing what to expect, the danger of
VBAC for the infant, the convenience of timing birth, and the
danger of VBAC for the mother.

Interestingly, the medical risks of uterine rupture to mother and baby associated with VBAC were very low on the women's lists of reasons for choosing cesarean section. And, similar to the findings of other studies discussed in these pages, the women seemed most concerned about protecting their expectations and gaining control over the situation but believed that medically, nothing would go wrong. In other words, many didn't expect to be able to deliver vaginally, so they didn't want to take the risk of disappointing themselves. They could expect to avoid labor pain with a cesarean, but they couldn't expect to avoid it with a VBAC. And they knew what to expect from surgery, so they weren't going to be disappointed by the unknown territory of VBAC.

A couple of other interesting points emerged from this study. Though the majority of patients at both hospitals were white, those from Hospital B were more highly educated and had most of their prenatal care in private offices, while those from Hospital A tended to have their prenatal care at a resident or county clinic, and only half attended their first prenatal visit in the first trimester. Of the women who responded to the questionnaires, 82 percent of Hospital A patients planned to attempt a VBAC, as opposed to only 55 percent of the Hospital B patients. The better educated women with more consistent prenatal care were less enthusiastic about VBAC. This may suggest that physicians at Hospital A were able to exert more influence over the less-educated patients there.

Second, the authors devote less than a single paragraph in the study to the 25 patients whose VBAC attempt failed, a total of 23 percent of those who tried. The authors state that 48 percent of these women said "they would never try VBAC again," while 20 percent said "they would definitely try VBAC again." They do not say how the other 32 percent felt. And, unlike the New York study, this study did not encompass how all of the women felt about their experiences afterward.

At Ochsner Foundation Hospital in New Orleans in 1989, the authors of the aforementioned Louisiana study, called "Vaginal Birth After Cesarean Section: The Impact of Patient Resistance to a Trial of Labor" set out to determine whether patient or physician resistance accounted for decisions in favor of repeat cesarean.

Of an initial group of 167 women with previous cesareans, 143 were eligible VBAC candidates. Of these, 51 attempted a VBAC and 35 succeeded. (Five of these 35 had planned a repeat cesarean but went into early labor, at which point the obstetrician was able to "change the patient's mind in favor of VBAC.") Of the 92 women who chose a repeat cesarean, 52 were VBAC-resistant patients, and the other 40 represented obstetrician resistance to VBAC. The reasons patients cited for declining a trial of labor included fear of labor, convenience of scheduled delivery, and fear of recurrent outcome (ending up with another cesarean). During the course of some of the pregnancies, both patients and obstetricians changed their minds about the preferred method of delivery. In summary, 36 percent of the resistance to VBAC was patient-directed, and 28 percent was physician-directed.

The study's authors suggest that the physician resistance was excusable. "Undoubtedly, had all of the 40 patients been subjected to a trial of labor, some of these patients may have been delivered vaginally," they write. "We remain convinced, however, that most of these patients would have labored unsuccessfully and feel supported in this belief by the birth weights."

They are less forgiving of the patients who resisted VBAC of their own accord (and do not report the birthweights of their babies). "These patients apparently view repeat cesarean delivery as an advantageous procedure that allows a known time of delivery without the uncertainties of attempted VBAC," they write. "Medical concerns pertaining to costs and safety seem to be overlooked by such patients." The inference is clear to me: These women behaved irresponsibly by taking the convenient, easy way out, which also happens to be the more expensive option. (Doctors can do that, but apparently not patients.) Furthermore, the women deliberately neglected their safety and the safety of their baby.

Without showing much interest in the reasons their patients cited for refusing a trial of labor, the authors conclude with the following chilling statement: "In our opinion, enhanced patient education and neutralization of the convenience factor should theoretically reduce patient resistance to a trial of labor in the future. Perhaps this type of approach would be preferable to a protocol of mandated trial of labor." What they mean by "enhanced patient education" or "neutralization of the convenience factor" is anybody's guess.

The Cost Issue

The current debate about how to curb escalating health care costs is beyond the scope of this book. With regard to childbirth, however, I believe cost should not be an issue that is imposed upon a woman when she is evaluating her birth options. Just as we don't limit the number of children people can have, which would really save the system money, we can't mandate one type of delivery over another for cost reasons alone. If a woman feels morally obligated to contribute to cost-cutting, she may choose the option that is mostly likely to cost less. And though the tab for vaginal birth typically runs less than for cesarean birth, there are no guarantees that a VBAC trial will cost less than an elective repeat cesarean. If other considerations are more important to the prospective mother and her partner, those should prevail.

A doctor who routinely performs cesarean sections to make more money is abusing the system, and some insurance companies are now compensating physicians equally for vaginal and cesarean deliveries, which is a step in the right direction. A woman who chooses a repeat cesarean, however, is not doing so to take something away from someone else; she is doing it because she believes it is best for the well-being of her baby and herself.

A letter from Dr. James R. Scott of Salt Lake City immediately following the Louisiana study makes several interesting points.

It would have been helpful, he writes, to provide more details on why the patients refused a trial of labor. "Were the women with a fear of labor or recurrent outcome those who had long, painful labors, poor outcomes, or complications associated with their labors that resulted in the previous cesarean section?" he asks. "In my experience these often have been factors."

Dr. Scott also asks whether the study's authors solicited any feedback from patients who ended up with another cesarean after a failed trial of labor, which he describes as "an interesting group of patients that have received little attention in most publications on VBAC." He describes two of his own patients' deliveries to illustrate these points.

The first patient gave birth by cesarean two weeks post–due date to a baby weighing 4000 grams (8 lbs. 13 oz.) She had a long, difficult, and eventually arrested labor. "She did not want to go through that again," writes Dr. Scott, and he believed that the baby she was carrying in the next pregnancy would also be large. This woman had a routine and uncomplicated repeat cesarean section one week before her due date, again delivered a 4000-gram baby, was discharged from the hospital in three days, and had a hospital bill of $2,408.

The second patient had her first cesarean section because her baby was breech. She preferred a repeat cesarean, and she wanted her tubes tied after the delivery (which can be done during the cesarean surgery), but Dr. Scott persuaded her to try a VBAC. This woman had an arduous second labor with many vaginal exams, pushed for more than two hours, and had to have a repeat cesarean because the baby's head remained too high in the pelvis. The baby was fine, but the woman developed a fever and an infection and was hospitalized for nine days, for a hospital bill of $5,806.

"In other words," Dr. Scott writes, "the patient that I persuaded to attempt a trial of labor failed after about 24 hours of labor, was in the hospital three times as long, and had a hospital bill more than twice as high as that of the patient who had a repeat cesarean section. Which patient do you think was happiest with her management?" Dr. Scott obviously cares about patient satisfaction. Is this too much to expect of all obstetricians?

Doctors are not gods, and even though the odds may favor VBAC in most situations, odds are not gods either. Going through labor is a nerve-wracking experience for many women. One strategy midwives employ is to work closely, side by side and head to head, with laboring mothers to help them relax as much as possible. For someone who is committed to VBAC, this may help. However, someone who faces another labor against her will, with a great deal of trepidation, is not likely to relax simply because her doctor tells her the odds of success or gives her a drug and then leaves the room. Many doctors pay lip service to the idea of patient support, but where are they when the hesitant, anxious, fearful laboring woman needs it most? Extra support is not routinely given or offered for women attempting a trial of labor after a cesarean section.

An Anthropologist's Study of VBAC

One researcher who has paid more attention than most to the reasons women choose VBAC or repeat cesarean is anthropologist Carol Shepherd McClain, Ph.D., of the University of California San Francisco. In 1983, several years before VBAC was being promoted in progressive U.S. institutions, McClain and helpers conducted interviews with 100 women in the Bay Area who had delivered a baby by cesarean, were pregnant again, were medically fit for VBAC, and knew trial of labor was an option.

In one article McClain published about her research, she shows how women formed decisions based largely on their own reconstruction of the previous cesarean section, and then selectively used medical information from their physicians to justify their decision. It's not that they didn't listen to their physicians, but that they also had their own agendas. "They selected pieces of communications from their current caretakers—residents, staff obstetricians, nurse-midwives—that reinforced their pre-existing preferences," she writes in the journal *Social Science and Medicine*.

McClain loosely stratifies the women into two groups that reflect personal ideologies and cultural models. One group, to which she says the majority belong, accepts pregnancy and childbirth as "medical events." This acceptance is a fairly recent development resulting from what she describes as the "medico-technological imperative of reproductive care that relies as heavily on enthusias-

tic and appreciative consumers as on expert practitioners." As examples of this imperative, she cites procedures that enable infer-
tile couples to have babies, others such as amniocentesis that
allow for prenatal diagnosis of defective fetuses, and of course,
cesarean section, which "corrects for biological deficiencies and
failures that cannot be controlled by other means."

Women who espouse the medical imperative, she says, not only
accept cesarean birth, they may prefer it, especially after having
gone through it once. "Some of the women in this study were
relieved by their prior cesareans," she writes, "and, in postpartum
interviews, by their repeat cesareans—both of which they viewed as
having rescued the fetus from some menace, usually brought about
by their own maternal deficiencies: a pelvic distortion, an ineffec-
tive labor, fetal hypoxia from lack of oxygen through a placental
failure, fetal asphyxia from a cord around the neck, and so forth."
For these women, she writes, cesarean section "does not represent
loss of control over one's own body" but rather is "the best way
to have a baby because it is easy, fast, can be scheduled, and because physicians are good at it . . . . Cesarean section in this view
also improves on nature by saving the mother from discomfort, in-
convenience, and exhaustion [although many women experience
all of these prior to the cesarean], and by saving the fetus from
being battered and bruised in its passage through the birth canal."

As someone who can relate to this definition fairly closely, I
can honestly say that cesarean section isn't just the preferred
method for some of us and our babies; it can become the only
viable method, and our children wouldn't be here without it.
However, while there is certainly a group of women who feel
shamed and inadequate after having a cesarean, I don't agree that
all of us attribute our cesareans to maternal deficiencies or blame
ourselves. Carrying a large baby, for instance, or having a baby
with the cord wrapped around its neck, does not resonate "maternal deficiency" to me any more than having freckles and brown
hair does.

Unfortunately, many women have been conditioned to believe
they have failed somehow if they don't deliver vaginally. For others, simply having a healthy baby in the end is what matters most.

The second group of women McClain describes are more leery of medical technologies and see them as "a compromise to ensure safety, something to avoid if possible, to accept under professional (expert) counsel." These are women who prefer midwives, birthing rooms and early discharge, or birth centers or home birth; they question routine procedures such as ultrasound and electronic fetal monitoring. Within this group is a smaller subgroup of women who avoid hospitals and doctors altogether in favor of home birth. These women assign a high value to complete personal control over childbirth, coupled with—and McClain doesn't come out and say this—an apparent implicit belief that their body is made for giving birth, less intervention is better, and nature meant for it to be this way.

Naturally, these women prefer VBAC to repeat cesarean, and for them, McClain writes, "vaginal birth was not a means, but an end in itself, a virtue, a once-in-a-lifetime experience not to be missed." These, women, too, associate cesarean section with failure, and feel they have to earn their place as mothers by overcoming the challenge of labor and proving they can deliver vaginally.

In another article, in *Culture, Medicine and Psychiatry*, McClain questions the long-held assumption that women's decisions are shaped primarily by their doctor's recommendations and the medical information they receive. In her study, for example, only 4 of the 100 women interviewed said that their doctors were the sole influence in their decision, although their recommendations were certainly important. Also important, however, are the social pressures that shape women's decisions about childbirth—relationships with partners, child-care responsibilities, work plans, and future childbearing plans. The issue of controlling escalating health care costs didn't come up in the study.

Following are some common characteristics of women in McClain's study who chose a trial of labor:

- Quick recovery was particularly important to these women, because they were in the position of having to care for two children immediately upon returning home from the hospital. They believed that recovery from a vaginal birth would be easier and faster.

- These women tended to have more negative feelings about their first cesarean than the women choosing repeat cesarean.

- Some felt their husbands would appreciate their "courage and strength" better if the husbands participated in a "natural" vaginal delivery.

- Some wanted to protect their husbands from having to watch a cesarean.

Characteristics of women who elected repeat cesarean included the following:

- The women had not had trouble recovering from their first cesarean and did not anticipate problems recovering from the second.

- One woman chose repeat cesarean even though she wanted to attempt a VBAC because she didn't think her husband could provide "the support she needed to succeed."

- Some wanted to protect their husbands from having to watch them go through a long and exhausting labor.

- Of the 56 women who had repeat cesareans, 22 also had their tubes tied at the same time (as opposed to only 4 of 44 delivering vaginally.)

The other major point McClain makes is that women tried to maximize their control over uncertainty. For instance, some only chose a trial of labor if their doctors agreed to let them end it if they desired. One woman with two prior cesareans agreed to attempt a trial of labor only if she went into labor spontaneously before her scheduled date for the elective cesarean, and if she then dilated quickly, and if the doctors promised to perform a cesarean at her request. This woman had not dilated sufficiently in her previous pregnancies and doubted that she would the third time.

McClain also found some women who wanted social recognition for having tried vaginal birth or having committed to it but were relieved when it didn't work out and they could avoid labor (for instance, in the event the baby was breech). It seems these women felt the need to prove something to someone other than themselves, and having an elective repeat cesarean without first saying they would try labor made them feel inadequate.

Unfortunately, though McClain mentions that she assayed maternal satisfaction and asked her respondents to compare their birth experiences, this information has not been published.

Informed Consent

If you have a trusting relationship with your doctor or midwife, one in which mutual respect prevails, you shouldn't have to resort to the "informed consent" principle to protect yourself and your rights as a patient. Unfortunately, most women don't know they even have such rights.

"A big weakness in childbirth education programs is a lack of information on women's rights and informed consent," says Nicette Jukelevics, M.A., a parent education coordinator in Torrance, California, and past chair of the International Childbirth Education Association's cesarean options committee. "I have found that to be an important tool for empowering women to get the birth they want and to avoid unnecessary interventions."

Most, if not all, states have a version of informed consent as a legal doctrine. At the very minimum, informed consent requires that before a provider touches you or performs a procedure, you have a right to have your questions about the risks and benefits of the procedure and its alternatives answered, and you have a right to say no.

Medical caregivers who follow ACOG's guidelines on informed consent to the letter will put considerably more effort into their relationship with you, making you an equal partner in the decision-making process as much as possible, from the start of prenatal care to the grand finale of delivery.

The eight-page ACOG committee opinion entitled "Ethical Dimensions of Informed Consent" is an eye-opening, patient-friendly document underscoring the importance of ethical integrity and disclosure in physician-to-patient communication. Although it does not specifically address the issue of choice with regard to VBAC or repeat cesarean, here are three enlightening passages:

- "Informed consent is an expression of respect for the patient as a person; it particularly respects a patient's moral right to bodily integrity, to self-determination regarding sexuality and reproductive capacities, and to the support of the patient's freedom within caring relationships."

- "Informed consent not only ensures the protection of the patient against unwanted medical treatment, but it also makes possible the active involvement of the patient in her or his medical planning and care."

- "The ethical concept of 'informed consent' contains two major elements: *free consent* and *comprehension* (or understanding) . . . . As 'free,' consent implies a choice between alternatives. It includes the possibility of choosing otherwise—as the result of deliberation and/or identification with different values and preferences. Free consent, in other words, implies the possibility of choosing this or that option or the refusal of any proposed option."

If there is any question in your mind or your caregiver's about ACOG's position on your right to choose between VBAC and repeat cesarean, here are the final lines from ACOG's 1994 committee opinion "Vaginal Delivery After a Previous Cesarean Birth": "Actions or policies that coerce patients to undergo either a trial of labor or a repeat cesarean procedure interfere with patient autonomy and the physician-patient relationship and undermine informed consent. The mode of delivery ultimately should be based on the specific clinical circumstances and the patient's choice after appropriate counseling."

Hospitals also have informed-consent documents but chances are you will first see one and be asked to sign it when you arrive, possibly in active labor. This is sort of a legalistic joke. Unless you have plenty of time on your hands and a hospital representative is present to explain every detail of such a form, you are not going to become very informed while you are doubled over with labor contractions. And if they say, sorry, we can't admit you until you sign this form, what are you going to do, leave?

One strategy is to obtain the form ahead of time, possibly when you tour the labor and delivery ward, and discuss any objections you might have with your own caregiver. In the event your own caregiver can't attend your delivery, and even if he or she does, you may want to bring several copies of your birth plan (see Chapter 6) to the hospital with you and give them to people who are assigned to take care of you. The most important thing is to know ahead of time which procedures and interventions are routinely used at your hospital and to tell your caregiver if you object to any of them. Fight your battles ahead of time so you don't waste precious energy fighting them during labor. Just in case something surprising comes up, though, even if you do sign the hospital's form, you can still change your mind about a procedure and say no to it later.

Informed consent is a controversial issue among doctors and subject to interpretation. Some doctors will deliberately inform patients more than others. Doctors are not paid to take extra time to explain a complex procedure or all the possible side effects of a drug. If a doctor feels strongly that procedure A is preferable to procedure B, he or she may not say much at all about procedure B.

In the past, doctors didn't give a woman with a prior cesarean the choice of attempting a trial of labor in her next pregnancy, following instead the edict "once a cesarean, always a cesarean." This is because the medical community itself was not informed enough about the risks of vaginal birth after cesarean and didn't consider it safe. Today, however, it can be argued that a doctor who doesn't discuss VBAC with patients and tells them carte blanche that they must have a repeat cesarean is violating informed-consent rules.

Conversely, some pro-VBAC doctors of late have been arguing that a woman doesn't get to choose elective cesarean section her first time, so there's no good reason she should have that choice during the next pregnancy. This is a specious argument on several counts:

- Whether it is reasonable or not to allow the choice of elective cesarean the first time is a separate ethical issue and not without controversy. A *New England Journal of Medicine* article, "Prophylactic Cesarean Section at Term?" (1985), used a hypothetical statistical model to show that elective cesarean at term would undeniably "save some babies destined for disaster." The paper pointed out that maternal death rates for elective cesarean are considerably lower than for nonelective cesarean and argued that for pregnant women belonging to a group with a primary nonelective cesarean rate of 27 percent or higher, elective cesarean may be a safer bet than a wait-and-see approach. "In light of all these considerations," the authors conclude, "is it tenable for us to continue to fail to inform patients explicitly of the very real risks associated with the passive anticipation of vaginal delivery after fetal maturity has been reached? If an informed patient opts for prophylactic [protective] cesarean section at term, can it be denied?"

- Though it is impossible to guess how many women would opt for elective primary cesarean section if allowed to choose, I suspect it would be nowhere near the 40 to 50 percent who currently opt for repeat cesarean section when given the choice. To mandate that all women with a prior cesarean have a trial of labor presumes that women are not capable of making a reasonable choice in collaboration with their caregiver.

- A VBAC labor comes with the additional risk of uterine rupture, which is not a risk in normal vaginal deliveries.

How could it be considered ethical to force a woman to undergo a VBAC trial if she chooses not to take that specific risk?

- If informed consent allows you to refuse the surgical intervention of a cesarean, does it then not also allow you to refuse the operative intervention of forceps, or the use of Pitocin to induce or augment labor, or the cutting of an episiotomy, all of which are associated with vaginal deliveries?

The bottom line is that you have a right to a reasoned dialogue with your caregiver about any question or alternative you wish to discuss. If your caregiver refuses to discuss or grant you a request that seems reasonable to you, such as a request for an epidural or a request not to have Pitocin, you can and should find another who will. But of course you cannot willingly change caregivers in the middle of labor, so it is essential to work these details out ahead of time and then bring your preferences in writing to give to the other attendants at the hospital.

More Support for Laboring Women

Some researchers have suggested that increased patient support would help to increase the VBAC rate. But what kind of support are they talking about, who gives it, and who pays for it? Imagine having a skilled female labor companion—someone who has given birth herself, someone in addition to your partner—who stays with you during the entire course of labor and helps you through it, physically and emotionally, and who explains everything that is happening and who does not leave the room in the middle of a painful contraction to let machines do the monitoring.

If you think having such a person (called a *doula*) present would ease some of your anxiety and help you look more favorably on a VBAC trial, you may be able to negotiate for it. It will probably cost you about $200 extra, but if you are straddling the fence with regard to a trial of labor, it may really help to have the additional support and advocacy that a doula can provide.

Just as nurse-midwife care is associated with a reduced cesarean rate, so is regular obstetric care augmented with a doula. An impressive study by John Kennell, M.D. and others in the *Journal of the American Medical Association* conducted in Houston showed significant differences in the labors and outcomes between three groups of about 200 women each.

Four hundred women admitted to Jefferson Davis Hospital in Houston were randomly assigned to either a doula-supported group or a neutral observer group. A third group of 200 women, who met the same criteria as the others, was assigned as the control group after delivery.

The doulas were women ranging in age from 22 to 55 who had experienced a vaginal delivery with a good outcome, who spoke English and Spanish fluently, and who went through a three-week training program in which they learned to distinguish between normal and abnormal labor, how to support laboring women, and which obstetric procedures the hospital was most likely to use.

After obtaining informed consent from the laboring patient to have the doula present, the patient met the doula for the first time upon being admitted. The doula stayed at her patient's side through delivery, "soothing and touching her patient and giving encouragement." She explained procedures, translated when necessary, and kept a written record of all hospital staff contacts, interventions, and procedures.

Women assigned to the neutral observer group simply had a person present through labor and delivery who kept a record of staff contacts, interventions, and procedures. The neutral observer did not speak to the laboring woman and did not get involved in the proceedings. Women in the control group received the hospital's standardized obstetric care, which is explained in detail in the study.

Some interesting differences in the three groups are:

- The cesarean rate was lowest for the doula group (8 percent), followed by the neutral observer group (13 percent) and the control group (18 percent). There were no fetal deaths. The control group had the highest proportion of cesareans for "failure to progress," but the numbers of cesareans for other indications, including fetal distress and cephalopelvic disproportion, were similar in the three groups.

- Although all three groups received narcotic painkillers in equal measure, the doula group had the lowest rate of epidural anesthesia (7.8 percent), followed by the neutral observer group (22.6 percent) and the control group (55.3 percent). The doula group also received epidurals later in the labor progression than the control group.

- The use of Pitocin to augment labor was lowest in the doula group (17%) and highest in the control group (43.6%). Pitocin was also administered later in the doula group and earlier in the control group. The women in the doula group had the shortest labors, and those in the control group the longest.

- Fewer babies born to doula-supported women remained in the hospital for more than 48 hours (10.4 percent), as opposed to 17 percent in the observer group and 24 percent in the control group. The rate of maternal fever was also lowest in the doula group.

The authors of the study speculate that some of the differences in outcomes between the neutral observer group and the control group could be because the observer's presence may have led staff members to follow hospital procedures more closely (for instance, to delay the administration of Pitocin and epidural anesthesia). It is possible, also, that the observer's presence acted as a conscience and led to more active patient support on the part of the staff.

It should be pointed out that the women served in this study (and this hospital in general) were low income and low educated (fewer than ten years of school), and few attended prenatal classes. More than half of the women in each group were single, and their average age was barely twenty. It is possible that this population can benefit more from doula support than an older, more educated and informed group of women. However, the presence of doulas within one homogenous sample of women clearly had a positive effect on outcome.

And the authors include an interesting discussion that relates to all laboring women about the correlation other studies have found between the laboring mother's anxiety level, measured by blood levels of stress hormones called catecholamines, and the decrease of uterine contractions. Animal studies, in addition, have shown that a reduction of blood flow to the uterus and placenta resulting in fetal distress is related to increased catecholamine levels.

"Thus, a supportive companion may reduce catecholamine levels by reducing maternal anxiety and facilitating uterine contractile activity and uterine blood flow," write the authors. "A *doula* may decrease maternal anxiety by her interactions with the laboring woman—her constant presence, physical touch, reassurance, explanations, and anticipatory guidance. These aspects of *doula* support may make the laboring woman feel safer and calmer, needing less obstetric intervention for labor to proceed smoothly."

As the authors conclude, "While there may be financial savings, the physical and emotional benefits of *doula* support for the welfare of mothers and infants make a compelling case for the review of current obstetric practices."

It would be interesting to see researchers test the doula hypothesis on women attempting VBAC. Take a large enough sample of women attempting VBAC in one hospital and randomize them into two groups, one with a doula and one without. My guess is this: not only would the doula group have a higher success rate, but these mothers would probably feel more satisfied with their overall birth experience, even if it resulted in a repeat cesarean. Maybe the hands-on support that overly busy doctors cannot provide is one thing more women could use to help them have a positive VBAC experience.

For women who are interested in doula support, good sources of information about these birth attendants and where to find one include childbirth education classes; local La Leche League meetings (though this organization does not refer women to specific doulas, other women attending the meetings may have recommendations); certified nurse midwives, who may work in tandem with doulas; flyers at obstetricians' offices; and local newspapers, in which doulas advertise. A sample of the quarterly magazine, *The Doula,* which publishes an article by a doula in each issue, can be ordered for $4.00 by calling (800)-MYDOULA or writing to P.O. Box 61, Santa Cruz, CA 95063.

The VBAC rate has risen each year, from just 6.0 percent in 1985 to 25.4 percent in 1993. As more physicians offer it and more women choose it, it is likely that the rate will continue to rise, though how much is difficult to predict. This is a good trend and should be allowed to continue on a natural course, without coercion on the part of insurance companies or overly zealous doctors.

A growing number of women want to try a VBAC, and with the collaboration and support of their doctors, and under the appropriate medical circumstances, they should be encouraged to exercise that choice. Another group of women who have experienced one or more cesareans prefer a repeat cesarean, which is not an unreasonable choice. Instead of being pressured, they, too, should be allowed to exercise that option and not be ostracized for doing so.

Finding the Right Medical Partner

When I was pregnant with my second child in 1992, I faced a difficult decision. My first baby had been born in 1988 at Northwestern Memorial Hospital, a top teaching institution in Chicago. He was delivered by a talented and caring obstetrician who did everything in her power to promote a vaginal birth. I had finally gone into labor two weeks late, the same morning I was scheduled for an induction. During the next eighteen hours, I never had regular contractions. They would spike up on the computer printout, along with the intensity of my pain, and then spike up again, not abating for several minutes. I never found a rhythm in labor and rarely got a break. After fourteen hours of this dysfunctional labor (the medical term), I had dilated to 6 centimeters.

My doctor consulted one of her older colleagues, who marched in authoritatively and, without as much as a hello, examined me with unusual force and ruptured my bag of waters. "Get a sump pump in here!" he yelled. "I've never seen so much water in my life!" He left and didn't return. (While it may have seemed funny to others at the time, at my expense, this was the sort of behavior that later made me want to have complete control over who delivered my next baby.)

My doctor tried to move things along with Pitocin, but the baby's heart rate kept taking nosedives. When the heart rate stayed down too long, a sudden swarm of attendants in the room began prepping me for an emergency cesarean section. But after a

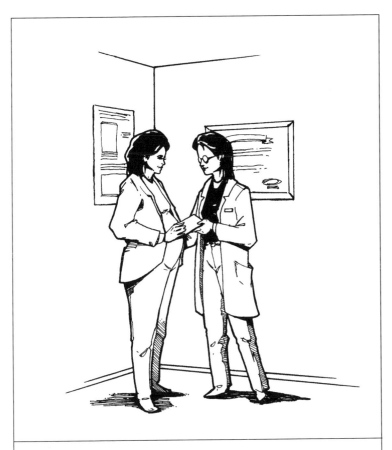

Choosing the Right Caregiver

Whether you prefer a VBAC or a repeat cesarean, finding a medical partner who will listen and respect your wishes is one of the most important choices you will make in your pregnancy.

couple of them lifted me and turned me in midcontraction and slapped an oxygen mask on my face, the heart rate bounced back up, and my husband, who had been kicked out of the room, was allowed back in.

Shortly before the pregnancy, I had served as the journalist for a climbing expedition to Mt. Everest in Nepal. I trekked for sixteen days from 6400 to 18,000 feet and camped on the glacier at the Everest base camp for six weeks, filing weekly stories with a portable computer. My team was ultimately driven off the mountain by one of the worst blizzards of the century before anyone could reach the summit. After that experience, I felt that I could tackle almost any new challenge.

During this labor, however, I began to lose my strength and composure. Mostly, I worried about the little life inside of me. I was trying hard not to think about the traumatic stillbirth my brother and his wife had experienced four years earlier.

I asked for and got an epidural. The contractions continued spiking irregularly with intermittent drops in the baby's heart rate. Four long hours passed, and I didn't dilate any further.

At the eighteen-hour mark, when my doctor said "I think it's time to get this baby out," I was relieved.

Except for the two anesthesiology residents who gabbed incessantly about the impending World Series next to my head and initially ignored my pleas for help when I started to gag and shake uncontrollably on the operating table, I had no complaints about the cesarean delivery. My husband was there and brought me the baby almost immediately. Additionally, I had developed a uterine fibroid early in the pregnancy, and though she had planned on leaving it alone, my doctor removed it because she thought it would cause problems later on. I felt lucky about that.

My son weighed 4445 grams (9 lbs. 13 oz.). Though pelvic sizes vary, I am only 5'6" tall and weigh 130 to 135 pounds. His large head (14.5 inches around) had been positioned asymmetrically in the birth canal. His Apgar scores were 8 and 9. I stayed in the hospital five days, which I needed; the baby nursed without any problems, and both of us recovered terrifically from the ordeal.

I could not go back to my obstetrician for my second pregnancy. My insurance had changed, and I had to see someone in the HMO network. Based on a recommendation from my primary care physician, I chose a younger woman on the Northwestern faculty. She was on maternity leave with her second child during my first two visits, so I saw other members of her practice.

When I met this doctor, she cheerfully pronounced me a perfect candidate for a VBAC. I had had a low transverse uterine incision, I was in excellent physical shape, and chances were the indications for the first cesarean—arrest of labor and fetal macrosomia—would not reoccur.

I was very unsure, however. There was no doubt in my mind that the cesarean had saved the baby's life, and possibly mine. The thought of repeating that experience for the sake of a VBAC was much scarier to me than having a repeat cesarean, which was a known quantity. What if I had another large baby that wouldn't fit through the birth canal? What if I labored for a very long time, in a great deal of pain, and still had to have a cesarean? I shared these reservations with my doctor, and she listened intently, always responding to my concerns, always agreeing to give me a repeat cesarean if I insisted, but maintaining that she believed I could deliver vaginally. I wondered whether she would be encouraging me to attempt a VBAC if she had attended my first delivery. I respected her professional judgment, but I anguished over the decision.

It didn't help that I was getting mixed messages from other members of the practice. The male doctor who had initially examined me said that I had a narrow pelvic outlet, possibly too narrow to deliver vaginally. Another shrugged off my fears of a vaginal delivery—and her partner's assessment of my pelvic capacity—and bombarded me with statistics about the efficacy of VBACS. "I've delivered second babies vaginally that are even bigger than the first," she boasted. Frankly, I didn't care, and her blithe dismissal of my feelings annoyed me. I had no desire to deliver another 9- to 10-pound baby vaginally, and the statistics did not console me. I wanted someone who could empathize.

So I called my first doctor, a mother of two herself, and asked what she would do. "Whatever they say, it's up to you," she said. "I'd suggest you make a deal. Figure out what you can live with and have an endpoint in mind, say 41 weeks, and if you haven't delivered by then, schedule a cesarean."

The idea that I could negotiate with my obstetrician was somehow a revelation, and her advice turned out to be prescient and invaluable. Yes, I knew I could opt for a repeat cesarean. But if I were willing to try a VBAC, were there certain conditions that would make it less scary, less painful, more palatable—things that would give me the semblance of having at least a little control?

Toward the end of the pregnancy, my husband and I hashed out a plan with my doctor. I agreed to let nature take its course until the 41st week, one week past the due date. If I didn't go into labor by then, I'd let her try an induction, just once. No going home from the hospital and coming back later. I definitely wanted an epidural. If the induction and VBAC didn't work, I insisted that she deliver the baby herself by cesarean before she went home at the end of the day—that gave us twelve hours to work with. She would have preferred I wait until the end of the 42nd week, but I refused, because more than anything I feared having another large baby that wouldn't fit.

I knew that babies can gain as much as an ounce a day toward the end of a pregnancy and that second babies are often larger than first babies. I also knew that boys are often larger than girls, and I was having another boy.

My doctor and I had a friendly disagreement over the estimated size of the second baby. She thought he was considerably smaller than the first, but I didn't think so. An ultrasound measurement supported her estimate of about 7.5 pounds, but I knew (and said so) that both she and the ultrasound were wrong.

My due date passed. I went for the induction three days later at 5:30 on a Friday morning, which was when she and the hospital could accommodate me. My doctor and I had a friendly wager. "There's no way this baby is more than 8 pounds, 1 ounce," she said, smiling. "I bet he is," I replied nicely. "He's closer to 9 pounds."

With the induction, I dilated much faster than any of us expected. Unfortunately, I was having back labor (the back of the baby's head was bumping against my sacrum, causing excruciating pain), and the first epidural only worked on the left side of my body. Though I kept calling this to attention of everyone in the room, it seemed as if no one except my husband really believed me (my doctor wasn't there yet), and the young anesthesiologist had performed a disappearing act. No explanation was given for the problem, and nothing more was done to relieve the pain until the very end. But at least the contractions were regular, so I could rest in between, and they were easier to cope with psychologically because I was really dilating this time.

Finally, I received a second epidural, but not before the anesthesiologist apparently also gave me a narcotic, which I never asked for and only learned of later. At about the same time the second epidural took effect, I had dilated to 10 centimeters. But the electronic fetal monitor showed that the baby's heart rate was decelerating and not coming back up.

"Liz, we've got to get this baby out," my doctor announced suddenly. "I can either do a cesarean or use forceps, your choice."

"We've gotten this far, and I won't feel it now, so why don't you try the forceps," I replied just as quickly, a little unnerved by this development. She said she needed me to help by pushing. Though numbed, I was able to push, and the baby was born almost immediately—with the umbilical cord wrapped around his neck. He wasn't breathing, and his first Apgar score was just 3. My doctor said that he was being injected with a drug called Narcan to counteract the narcotic, which is how I learned I had received the narcotic and which explained why I could barely keep my eyes open. A team resuscitated him in a far corner of the room, and his 5-minute score rose to an 8.

My intuition about his size was correct: he weighed 8 pounds, 13 ounces. Had I waited until the 42nd week, he might have weighed about 9.5 pounds. I was glad I had insisted on the 41-week cutoff.

I suffered a cervical laceration and a third-degree vaginal laceration, thanks to the midforceps delivery. I had a large episiotomy and a case of hemorrhoids that felt like I had grown a tail. The recovery from these problems was long and painful. I had avoided major abdominal surgery and a long labor (the second one took seven hours). The hospital stay was three days shorter and the VBAC was less costly. Though I could get around and resume moderate exercise sooner than I had after my cesarean, the pain lasted much longer. The perineal area of my body has never been the same.

The VBAC worked, but it was hardly a cathartic experience for me (though it made my doctor very happy). I didn't feel any different about my body or about myself as a woman. Thankfully, the baby was okay, but the first Apgar score of 3 seemed pretty dicey to me. I almost ended up with a repeat cesarean at the last minute, and I would have been disappointed and angry had that occurred. On the other hand, I would have felt fine about an elective repeat cesarean. There are no guarantees, of course, but when your doctor tells you that you are a perfect candidate for a VBAC, you think it will probably work. But she doesn't know whether it will, and neither do you.

The most valuable thing I learned from my VBAC experience was the importance of the negotiating I had done. I am convinced the VBAC succeeded because I held my ground on issues like the timing. I wouldn't have agreed to try it otherwise. I had a good relationship with both of my doctors but more of a power struggle with the second one. As long as both parties listen and remain flexible, I think a power struggle is healthy, especially in cases like mine, where you are receptive to the idea of a VBAC but you also have real doubts and fears. It's important not to underestimate the power of your first birth experience, the power of any trauma you might have felt as a result of the cesarean. It's important not to let your caregiver dismiss your feelings about that experience.

Choosing a Caregiver

So how does my saga relate to yours? First, selecting a caregiver who will meet your individual needs is never more crucial than during pregnancy, which is exactly when many women feel most vulnerable. Whose baby is this after all? If you are a savvy consumer who wants a medical expert to work as your partner, not your superior, you need to show up to your prenatal visits with plenty of questions, the answers to which will help you decide what you would prefer and not prefer during pregnancy and labor. You have choices in childbirth, and they begin here.

If you are a VBAC candidate, the choice of caregiver is even more important. If you know what you want, at least you can look for someone whose philosophy matches yours. If you are clueless, the kind of person who typically answers, "Well, my doctor wants me to have . . . " when a friend asks what type of delivery you are hoping for next, you risk having that doctor impose his or her agenda on you, whether it's a repeat elective cesarean or a trial of labor. Are you willing to sacrifice your right to vote? If you are uncertain what to do, as I was, the best fit is someone who can help you decide by presenting the facts objectively, listening respectfully, and being flexible. My doctor met all of these needs.

Many of us are afraid to ask questions of doctors, especially obstetricians and gynecologists. We spend more time decorating the baby's room than searching for the most compatible person to help bring the baby into the world. Doctors can be formidable and make us feel small and uncomfortable. It doesn't foster the *mano a mano* rapport to have the doctor fully clothed and standing, talking down at you while you are lying naked below the waist with your feet in stirrups. (Imagine what *he* would feel like lying naked on the table with his feet in stirrups!)

Remember, you will be seeing this caregiver at least once a month for the next eight months, and once every week or two by the end of the pregnancy. It's better to find out early if you picked a lemon, when there is still time to switch. But avoiding a confrontation now over some disagreement and settling for someone who treats you with less respect than you deserve is a mistake.

Male or Female Obstetrician?

If you decide to go with an obstetrician, do you care whether your obstetrician is male or female? If you don't think it matters, you may want to read the national bestseller *Women and Doctors*, by John M. Smith, a former ob-gyn, which documents abuses against women by the male-dominated medical community in general and obstetricians and gynecologists in particular.

"I have had a colleague invite me to do an exam on one of his patients under the false guise of a consultation because 'she has a body you won't believe,'" writes Dr. Smith. "I have seen more than one gynecologist walk into an operating room where another doctor's patient was already asleep for surgery, lift up the sheet, admire the patient's breasts, and continue his conversation without pause." Doctors are people, and they have character flaws like the rest of us. As Dr. Smith points out, "if you send a sexist to medical school, you can only wind up with a sexist doctor. Nothing in the academic medical environment results in the restructuring of male attitudes and prejudices." If you feel uncomfortable exposing your body to an unfamiliar male, why do it? By choosing a female, at least you remove one element of potential risk that can result from a skewed male-female dynamic.

Another obvious argument in favor of a woman is her ability to bear children. Personally, it helped me to know that each of my obstetricians had been through childbirth herself, and for that reason, I felt they could be more empathetic in this situation than a man could and would view me with more than just a clinical approach. This may sound like reverse sexism to some, but I imagine that men would be more suited to treat a patient with prostate problems and that most males with prostate problems would prefer to be treated by a male.

However, it's also understandable to me why some males devote their careers to delivering babies. There is no human event more highly charged than the live birth of a wanted child (the tears flowed freely from my otherwise stoic, normally tearless husband), and what nobler service could someone perform than to usher a new life into the world? As some women attest, males can make great obstetricians.

"He's about the most mellow person in the world, not at all controlling," says Karen C. of Dr. Randall Toig, the obstetrician at Northwestern Memorial Hospital in Chicago who delivered all three of her children. "After I had a cesarean with the first, he asked what I wanted to do," she recalls. "I asked if he had any thoughts about it, and he said, 'Yeah, my thoughts are, what do you want to do?' I said I wanted a VBAC, and he said, 'That's great, then that's what we'll try to do.'" She was very pleased with his care and did indeed deliver her second and third children vaginally.

Ask friends whose judgment you trust for recommendations of caregivers, and ask what specifically they liked about their doctor.

If you are new to an area, try calling the maternity ward of a respected hospital and ask for names from the obstetrics nurses. If you are in an HMO, ask your primary care physician for specific names within a practice. Once you have a list, call the office of the first doctor, tell the receptionist you are pregnant and looking for a caregiver and would like to schedule an appointment to talk to the person, without being examined.

Screening the Doctor and the Hospital

If the receptionist insists that all first visits must include a pelvic exam, you may want to scratch this doctor from your list, write Diana Korte and Roberta Scaer, authors of *A Good Birth, A Safe Birth*. "If you go ahead with the exam first, one of two outcomes is likely: You will find changing doctors extremely difficult even if the one who examined you is not Dr. Right; or, after she's examined you, the doctor is more likely to become aggravated at your questions, your taking your time to make up your mind, or your decision to change doctors. Remember, you are negotiating first whether this person is Dr. Right." Also, as they note, a pelvic exam administered by a total stranger immediately puts you in a vulnerable position and may make you uncomfortable.

Then, says Korte, also author of *Every Woman's Body*, come prepared to the interview with a prioritized list of questions—for example, if having another person present at the delivery besides your husband is crucial, ask that first. Bring someone, such as your husband or a good friend, along to the appointment to serve as another set of ears. Another tip from Korte: collect all the drugs and vitamins you are taking, toss them in a bag, and take them to the interview. It's a visual cue to the provider that you take your own health care seriously. Another thing I learned from my experience: not only should your doctor have a record of your prior obstetrics history, but it can be enlightening for you to get a copy of the delivery summary from your prior delivery. If it is not with your obstetrics records, the hospital should have a copy. The delivery summary provides many interesting details about the birth that may not have been communicated to you at the time. The purpose of this initial appointment is twofold: to get as many objective, straightforward answers as you can about policies and procedures; and equally if not more important, to assess this person as a human being.

One often-overlooked issue is the very real possibility that your own physician will not be there to deliver your baby. This is especially important if having a VBAC is your goal and if you are hashing out a specific plan with your own doctor. (If you are having an elective repeat cesarean, you will most likely be able to schedule it with your own doctor.) Will your plan go by the way-side if another member of the practice attends your delivery? It's important to find out how many of her own patients she delivers versus how many of her colleagues' patients. What is her call schedule? Does she deliver at more than one hospital? How many other doctors are in the practice? Can you meet them all? In short, do their philosophies mesh with hers and yours?

"A good OB practice, whether it's two or 22, recognizes that this is a major issue and sets up things so it works," says Dr. Smith. "When a physician says your wishes will be respected, he should mean anybody who happens to be there will respect them. One way is to see each of a group who might be on call and if you find one is thoroughly obnoxious, make that known, and that's another negotiating point."

Another important point, of course (and again, this should extend to all the members of the practice), is the doctor's position on cesarean sections in general. You may ask a doctor's cesarean rate, but this doesn't tell the whole story, since one doctor may see more high-risk patients than another. In the 1994 Public Citizen's Health Research Group report, *Unnecessary Cesarean Sections: Curing a National Epidemic*, the authors Mary Gabay and Sidney M. Wolfe, M.D. suggest that doctors with high-risk practices should have cesarean rates no higher than 17 percent, while those with low-risk practices should have rates under 10 percent. These figures provide an interesting index or point of comparison, but the high figure may be artificially low, since the national cesarean rate was still 22.8% percent in 1993. A doctor who sees primarily high-risk patients may in fact have a cesarean rate of 40 percent for good reason.

Like many consumer-advocate childbirth books, *Unnecessary Cesarean Sections* suggests that you find out your hospital's cesarean rate and poses a list of questions to ask a "hospital administrator." All well and good, but practically speaking, not very realistic. I put their advice to the test by calling the maternity ward of one notably progressive Chicago hospital and asking for one piece of information, the cesarean rate. I was shunted to eleven different people, back and forth between the medical records department, the maternity ward, media relations, even the financial services department, and still didn't get my answer. Though Massachusetts and New York have passed laws requiring hospitals to provide consumers with their cesarean rates, hospitals in general are as impenetrable as state and federal bureaucracies when it comes to divulging information. Besides, each is organized differently, and the phone book may or may not let your fingers walk to the right department.

You can save yourself some trouble by asking your doctor or midwife what the rates are. If they don't know, they should at least be able to tell you how to find out, since they will be more familiar with the hospital's unique structure and which department keeps track of such information. Easier still, but about $30 more expensive, you can order Public Citizen's 530-page book, which contains a state-by-state, hospital-by-hospital documentation of cesarean and VBAC rates. That allows you to compare your prospective hospital's rate with others in the area, especially if you live in or near a major metropolitan area.

Realistically, you will probably choose your doctor or midwife first, and your delivery will occur wherever that provider has admitting privileges. Talking to the provider should by extension answer most of your questions about how you will be treated at the hospital. On the other hand, a doctor may say it's fine with him if you have a doula or other labor companion besides your mate in attendance, but the hospital's policy may prohibit it. So, along with the list of questions you bring to the doctor, be sure to find out whom you can contact at the hospital to schedule a tour of the facility. Then, if there are unanswered questions after your doctor screening—such as the frequency of electronic fetal monitoring, which may depend more on hospital policy than doctor preference—you can save these questions for the tour.

If you are interested in a VBAC, instead of relying solely on a doctor's cesarean or VBAC rate, it may be more informative to ask specific questions. For instance, ask if the doctor will allow you to labor as long as your health and the baby's are not compromised, even if it means twenty-four hours or longer. Ask how many VBACs he has attended, and ask whether your labor and delivery will be handled differently because of your prior cesarean. If so, how and why? Note whether the doctor is enthusiastic about accommodating your wishes. If you want a VBAC, beware of any doctor who assigns a specific time limit on the length of labor—this could suggest that the doctor is overly concerned about missing tee-off time the next morning.

If you have given birth in a hospital once already, you know that the array of high-tech terms and technologies attached to childbirth in the United States is nothing short of mindnumbing. It will lower your intimidation index and elevate your level of power over the situation to familiarize yourself ahead of time with labor lingo and delivery room dialect.

Following are some other key questions to discuss and negotiate early. You can try to cover them all in your initial meeting, but in case time runs out, number them in order of their importance to you and remember to take notes. If you would like to make up a written birth plan, tell your doctor of your intentions at this meeting; afterward, document in writing everything you would prefer in labor and delivery. You can give it to her at your next appointment, provided this is the doctor you want. If you think you may want to revise it from time to time, wait to give it to her closer to your due date. Make sure any other doctor in the practice who might attend also has a copy, as well as your partner, other labor companion, and one for yourself at the hospital. This helps to ensure that there are no misunderstandings about the points you have worked hard to negotiate in advance. It sends a clear message that you are taking an active role in the decisions about your pregnancy, labor, and delivery experience.

Questions about pregnancy:

- For which patients do you recommend amniocentesis or chorionic villus sampling (two different tests for detecting fetal abnormalities)?

- Do you perform routine ultrasounds, and if so, how often and for what reasons?

- I would like to continue with my exercise program. What are your thoughts on this?

- I have a preexisting condition (such as pollen allergies) for which I regularly take medication. Are you going to tell me I have to stay indoors and not take my medication? How can my need to have this medication be balanced with the risk it might incur to the fetus?

- What are your thoughts on weight gain?

Questions about labor and delivery:

- Does the hospital where you deliver routinely administer enemas or shaves?

- May I have my husband and a doula or another person in the labor and delivery room at all times, even if I have a cesarean section? (A doula is a trained labor companion who has given birth herself and who can provide a different kind of support than your partner.) Unless your partner is a health care professional, he or she may be overwhelmed by the changes you are experiencing naturally as well as the high-tech obstetric procedures. Doulas may decrease your anxiety and take pressure off your partner to be your sole advocate and comforter. See Chapter 5 for more on doulas.

- Will you let me decide if I want an epidural or other pain medication?

- Under what circumstances would you administer Pitocin?

- Under what circumstances would you break my bag of waters?

- Do you believe in continuous electronic fetal monitoring or IVs? If so, does the hospital have portable equipment so that I can move and walk during labor?

- Do you perform episiotomies routinely or just sometimes?

- May I see and modify the hospital's informed-consent document ahead of time so I don't have to worry about it when I arrive in labor? (If you sign a blanket consent form at the hospital, you are giving up certain rights to say yes or no to certain procedures. It is much safer to have the risks and benefits of each procedure explained individually.)

- Will the baby be given to me immediately after birth?

- Can the baby and my husband room in with me?

Bedside manner

As you are checking off some of the questions on your list, carefully evaluate the doctor's people skills as well.

"If you find a doctor who doesn't want to talk, because he has the attitude that he's in charge, I would strongly suggest finding another doctor," says Dr. Smith. If a doctor doesn't want to explain procedures or answer questions now, he will probably be even less forthcoming later on. Since there are many common elements to most pregnancies, it's easy for people providing the care to act like automatons. If your interviewee acts this way, if she isn't listening or making eye contact on the first visit, don't expect her to be any better the next time. Someone who listens patiently and responds thoughtfully to your questions now is probably going to treat you the same way during labor and delivery.

"I went for a gentle, nice person with a lot of skill," says Dr. Phyllis Marx, a Chicago-area obstetrician (and my medical advisor for this book) who had the advantage of observing a lot of doctors before she chose hers. "The thing that drew me to him was his bedside manner, his gentleness, his respect for people. A lot of physicians have a tendency to be so egotistical. The self seems to be what comes out, as opposed to 'what can I do for you?' Well, this is not what I picked."

In her own practice, which includes three other women and a midwife, Dr. Marx allots an hour for the first obstetric visit. "It doesn't take a lot of time to take time for people," she says. "Some doctors will argue with me and say what we do is become more inefficient by taking more time. If I spend the time initially to introduce people to things I think are important, they're better informed, they feel much more of a relationship with me, and they may need less time later on. They develop a trust, and they know it's okay to call. I think people are important, so I try to make them feel good about themselves."

Have You Considered a Midwife?

Another option that's becoming increasingly popular is having a nurse-midwife care for you. About 4.7 percent of American hospital births were attended by these professionals in 1993—the last year statistics were available.

A certified nurse-midwife (CNM) is a registered nurse with twelve to twenty-four months of extra training in pregnancy care, after which she must pass a national certification exam. CNMs must collaborate with a doctor, and many OB practices now have some on staff who deliver at the same hospital. Performance studies of CNMs reveal very favorable delivery outcomes for both mothers and babies, as well as a high degree of maternal satisfaction.

"My relationship with the midwife was much more of a partnership, and I felt I was respected as an individual who was participating rather than as a slab of meat who was talked about as though I wasn't even in the room," says Chicagoan Suzanne S., who was told by a nurse attending her first son's delivery that she couldn't push when she was ready because her obstetrician had just gone to dinner.

If you are committed to trying a VBAC, if you would like to have less high-tech intervention than you had the first time, and if you both agree that you are a low-risk patient (a prior cesarean shouldn't automatically label you high-risk, but you will need to work that out with her), you may find a good fit in a CNM. A brief policy statement by the American College of Nurse-Midwives supports the concept of VBAC and says that certified nurse-midwives are qualified to take care of women desiring a VBAC "if appropriate arrangements for medical consultation and emergency care are in place."

Most midwives are female, and their approach is considerably different from most physicians' approaches.

For one thing, they tend to spend more time with you at each monthly visit—about an hour—and they will ask questions about your whole health, not just your pregnant uterus. They will typically advise you to labor at home longer than an obstetrician would. Once they meet you at the hospital, they stay with you throughout your labor and delivery.

Midwives rely more on hands-on skills and use high-tech medical intervention—such as epidurals, episiotomies, IVs, Pitocin, and continuous electronic fetal monitoring—only when yours or the baby's health is at risk. They are more likely than an obstetrician to let labor continue indefinitely, as long as mother and child are doing fine.

On the other hand, they can't perform cesareans. Fewer births attended by them end up as cesareans, but this may be in part because they don't take on women identified as high-risk patients in the first place. Midwives are more likely to try to persuade a woman that her body will be able to give birth "naturally."

If you choose a certified nurse-midwife, you will have important questions to raise early on with her, too.

- Who is your backup physician? How quickly can he or she get there, and under what circumstances would you need to call for backup? How often have you needed to call a physician?

- If I need a cesarean, will you stay with me in the operating room?

- What is your philosophy about pain medication? If I decide I want an epidural, will you call in an anesthesiologist?

- In the birthing room, who has control over such matters as how, and how often, the baby's heart rate is monitored and how much I can move around?

Playing Your Part

While you may discuss your wishes at length with your doctor or midwife, you too have some responsibilities in developing a trusting relationship. The first is, don't tell the doctor or midwife how to do her job. If you are a professional, you would feel insulted and uncomfortable if someone who is not an expert in your field told you how to do your job. A doctor's job is to use the skills he or she has garnered from delivering many babies. Although asking her to explain her policies and hear your desires is vital, telling her how to handle a pregnancy and birth shows a lack of trust.

If you are planning to take an active negotiating role in your delivery, you also have a responsibility to educate yourself before you first meet with a doctor. That will help you intelligently discuss the issues that matter most. But be flexible. If you have decided to trust a person, try to accept her medical expertise when she disagrees with you.

"If somebody says she never wants pelvic exams, I can try to respect her wishes, but I can't promise," says Dr. Marx. "In medicine, nothing will be in black and white, and I may not always be able to keep that promise, but I will try my best."

The most difficult patient, says Dr. Marx, is the one whose ways are too set—the person, for example, who announces that her labor is going to take eight hours, that she will deliver vaginally no matter what, that she won't have an epidural, and that she can handle anything. "I spend more time telling people to come into this experience with an open mind and not to expect something to be a certain way, because they will surely be disappointed. It is usually not what you expect."

If you have done everything you can to educate yourself on your choices, to select the best provider, and to negotiate the birth you desire, you still may not get exactly what you want. But you will feel more empowered during the climactic birth experience, and probably calmer as well, because you will have a better idea of what's going on, what's next, and what to anticipate at each successive stage. And even if the birth doesn't turn out the way you scripted it, you can feel assured that you took every responsibility you could for the health of yourself and your baby.

PART TWO

. . . .

Mothers' Voices

· · · · · ·

Introduction to Part Two

You now know some of the views and motivations of the medical community, the insurance lobbies, and national policymakers on the drive to lower the cesarean rate and increase the number of VBACs. But you haven't heard much from parents of newborns, particularly other mothers.

As noted earlier, only a handful of studies have focused on how mothers interpret their childbirth experiences and on which factors from the previous experience they base their preferences for subsequent births. Little has been written specifically about how a woman's perceptions of her first cesarean experience influence her feelings and decisions about an attempted VBAC versus an elective repeat cesarean in her next pregnancy. This is, of course, colossally important. And all parties involved in trying to increase the VBAC rate might want to pay more attention to mothers if they truly care about enhancing the quality of the birth experience.

The medical community appears to care less about the satisfaction quotient than the objective outcome of childbirth; mothers care a great deal about both. Wouldn't it be helpful, for instance, to know why some women welcome the opportunity to attempt a VBAC while others clearly prefer an elective repeat cesarean? Wouldn't it be useful to know how women feel about their VBACS, unsuccessful VBACS, and elective repeat cesareans afterward?

To solicit answers to these and other questions, I developed two informal surveys. The VBAC Women Survey was sent to women who had had a VBAC (in some cases, more than one VBAC). The Repeat Cesarean Survey was sent to women who had had one or more repeat cesareans.

A total of fifty-one women filled out the surveys. One woman's Repeat Cesarean Survey was ineligible because she had

had a classical incision with her first cesarean and therefore did not have a true choice in her subsequent pregnancy--her repeat cesarean was considered the only reasonable medical option. (Some staunch VBAC proponents will disagree with this statement, despite the 12 percent risk of uterine rupture with a classical incision.) Four women qualified for more than one category: Amy of Santa Barbara, California had a VBAC followed by an unsuccessful VBAC attempt that resulted in a cesarean; Julia of Los Angeles and Charlene of Montclair, New Jersey both had an unsuccessful VBAC followed by an elective repeat cesarean; and Sandra of Oshkosh, Wisconsin didn't have the VBAC she wanted for baby number two and had two elective cesareans for babies number three and four. Thus, while there were fifty eligible participants, the number of post-cesarean experiences tallied was fifty-four. (A repetition of the same type of experience, such as two VBACs or two elective repeat cesareans, was only counted once.)

Because all of the women who responded had experienced a primary cesarean, the first nine questions of both surveys were identical. These first nine questions, reprinted in Chapter 7, sought factual information about the cesarean as well as the women's emotional responses to it. Chapter 7 further explores relationships that might exist between how women felt about the first cesarean and their subsequent preferences in the next pregnancy.

Chapter 8 focuses on the stories of the twenty-six women who had a VBAC. The ten additional questions posed to these women are reprinted in this chapter, along with the women's responses. They were asked, among other things, whether they preferred their VBAC to their first cesarean experience and whether they would try VBAC again if they had another child.

There were twenty-five women who had a total of 28 repeat cesareans. To qualify for this survey, a woman simply had to end up with a repeat cesarean; she could have elected to have a repeat cesarean, attempted a VBAC that resulted in a cesarean, or wanted to attempt a VBAC but didn't for some reason. As it turned out, there were sixteen cases of elective repeat cesarean and twelve cases in which women ended up with another cesarean after attempting a VBAC or wanting to attempt a VBAC. Chapter 9 focuses on the women who wanted to have a VBAC but couldn't, a group often ignored by the medical community, which calls this experience a "failed trail of labor." The nine questions posed to these women about their repeat cesarean are reprinted in this chapter.

Chapter 10 addresses the women who elected to have a repeat cesarean. They answered the same questions (10 through 18) as the group in Chapter 9.

As I am not a scientist, and as my sample size is small, I make no claims that the experiences or feelings of these fifty women represent a typical segment of the population of childbearing women. I found these women by calling people I knew (thereby already introducing a geographical as well as socioeconomic bias) and asking if they knew women who had had a VBAC or repeat cesarean. In many cases, women who were enthusiastic about the surveys graciously passed them on to their friends. One woman responded to a sign posted in a Chicago bookstore. One was referred by a midwife and one by a physician. In short, 50 other women divided into the same categories might have responded entirely differently. My aim was to capture a range of experiences, to take a snapshot of one group of women who have faced the VBAC option.

Though the actual range of experiences is surely wider than what fifty people can bring to the table, my hope is that women in the position to choose a trial of labor or a repeat cesarean will gain some perspective and insight from the shared experiences of others. Though you may not find anyone with an experience just like yours, I hope these stories can help clarify your position and feelings, especially if you are ambivalent. And for those of you who may know exactly what you want, I hope you find resonance and affirmation in the stories of others who have gone before.

. . . . . .

The First Cesarean

All fifty women who responded to either the VBAC Survey or the Repeat Cesarean Survey answered the same set of questions about their first cesarean experience.

First-Cesarean Questions

1. Mother's age at time of first baby's birth (assuming first birth was C-section) or first C-section.

2. Was the baby early, on time, or post due? How late?

3. Where did you deliver? (private for-profit or public hospital; urban or rural; teaching hospital) Was your doctor male or female, older (50+) or younger?

4. Why did you have a C-section? How far did you dilate? How long were you in labor? Were drugs (Pitocin) used to augment or induce labor? Were drugs used as painkiller (epidural, other)?

5. Did your doctor make every effort to promote a vaginal birth?

6. Do you feel your C-section was necessary for both your baby's and your well-being?

7. What was the condition of the baby at birth?

8. Did you have any problems recovering from the C-section? How long did you stay in the hospital?

9. Did you feel as if you had failed somehow? Or that you had trouble bonding with the baby because of the C-section?

Demographics

The average age of the fifty women at the time of their first cesarean was 30 years ±4.4 years. Most of the women (forty-two) delivered in a private hospital; the remaining delivered in a public hospital. Male physicians attended thirty-three deliveries, female physicians attended sixteen; one respondent didn't say whether the physician was male or female.

Reasons for the Cesarean

First, let's look at the reasons women gave for the primary cesarean in terms of their expressed preferences for the next pregnancy. (Since more than one reason was given in some cases, the total number of reasons adds up to more than fifty.)

Of the thirty-seven women who attempted or wanted to attempt a VBAC, the most common reason for the first cesarean was breech presentation. There were fourteen women in this group, including one who was carrying twins with the presenting baby in breech position. Eight of the fourteen had scheduled cesareans before labor; the other six labored, including three who dilated 8 to 10 centimeters before being sectioned (two had doctors who didn't realize the baby was breech until that point).

The second most common indication for the first cesarean was failure to progress (FTP), a group of thirteen women, including eight whose labor arrested at various stages (they stopped dilating) and five who dilated fully and pushed but whose baby didn't descend (arrest of descent). These five really wanted a VBAC, and all five were later successful.

The third most common indication for the first cesarean in the group that later attempted VBAC was fetal distress, numbering 9.

Three women, all of whom went on to have VBACs, had cesareans for maternal complications: one had a placental abruption, and one developed a fever and intrauterine infection (though the primary reason for her section was fetal distress). The third had developed toxemia in her sixth month. Upon being induced one week before her due date, she dilated fully and began pushing, when the doctors suspected her placenta had abrupted. Her cesarean was performed under general anesthesia. The baby was borderline low birthweight (5.5 pounds) but otherwise healthy.

Finally, one woman, Sandra of Oshkosh, Wisconsin, underwent her first cesarean for cephalopelvic disproportion. She delivered the first of four children in 1987 at the age of thirty-three. Early in the pregnancy, her doctor told her she had a small pelvic opening, which could preclude a vaginal delivery. "I put that out of my mind throughout the pregnancy," Sandra wrote.

Sandra went into labor ten days after her due date. About fifteen hours into her labor, when she had dilated to 5 centimeters, the doctor took an x-ray of her pelvis, "which clearly displayed a head overlapping my pelvic bone openings." Her cesarean was done under a general anesthesia (hospital policy at the time). The healthy baby girl weighed 8 pounds 12 ounces. Sandra could not breastfeed the baby the first night, but she was "finally alert enough to realize motherhood" twelve hours later.

Feeling that she had "failed myself and my husband" Sandra was certain she wanted to try a VBAC in her next pregnancy, two years later. She went to the same doctor, who was agreeable to a trial of labor, though he said he doubted she could deliver vaginally because he suspected the second child would be larger than the first. Sandra, her husband, and the doctor agreed to wait one week past her due date and then induce labor.

But the hospital had a policy that profoundly affected her decision. If she labored and ended up with a cesarean, it would be done under general anesthesia. An elective repeat cesarean, however, would be done with a spinal.

"What loomed as most important to me was being there, being aware, when my child was born," Sandra wrote. "That took precedence over wanting to try anything."

One week past her due date, she was not showing signs of going into labor, and her doctor now insisted that the baby would be larger than the first one. Sandra and her husband hashed it out some more and decided the most important things were, in order, the safety of the baby and being there and being a part of the birth. They decided to have the cesarean. "I cried for two hours and then said to myself, 'Let it go. Tomorrow I'll be there for my child's birth and if I focus on this not being a vaginal birth, I'll miss the joy of how extraordinary it all is.'"

She had a spinal, and she and her husband listened to rock and roll during the surgery and laughed and joked with the nurses. The healthy baby boy weighed 9 pounds 1.5 ounces. "It was one of the happiest days of my life," Sandra wrote. "There were no complications. In comparison to my first birth, I felt totally aware, no nausea, only minor drowsiness. I had free interaction with friends and family, and as much touching and holding and loving of my son as I desired. The method of anesthesia, for me, made all the difference."

Sandra had two more babies by elective repeat cesarean. She described the third birth as "perfect and fun" and the fourth as "wonderful."

Sandra's childbirth history might have unfolded differently if she were giving birth to the second baby today, less than ten years later. She would probably be offered an epidural in a VBAC trial, and the epidural would be used in the event a cesarean became necessary. This would have been the incentive she needed to attempt a trial of labor. Nobody knows, of course, what the outcome would have been. But Sandra made peace with herself about the first cesarean, which enabled her to delight in the births of her other three children.

There were sixteen women in the group who chose an elective repeat cesarean (thirteen did so in their second pregnancy and three in their third; see below). The most frequent reason for the first cesarean in this group was failure to progress.

Among the eight cases of FTP in the first pregnancy, one woman, Chris of Oak Park, Illinois, reported being in labor three days. Two and a half days into it, she was given a sedative to get some sleep. Then she was induced with Pitocin, but still only dilated 1 centimeter. Two other women labored twenty-four hours, and two more women labored fifteen to twenty-four hours. The sixth had dilated just 2 centimeters after ten hours.

Two of the women with FTP in their first pregnancy tried VBAC the second time and ended up with a repeat cesarean again for failure to progress. These two, Julie and Charlene, both opted to have elective repeat cesarean in their third pregnancies.

Four women in the elective-cesarean group had their first cesarean because of a breech presentation. There were three cesareans for cephalopelvic disproportion, including one in which a baby with congenital abnormalities died sixteen hours after birth. Two cesareans were done for fetal distress, including one in a woman carrying two fetuses, one of which had died in utero.

Was it Necessary?

The women's answers to questions 5 and 6 provide clues about whether they agreed with the doctor's decision to perform a cesarean and whether they felt the cesarean was justified.

Three fourths of the fifty women answered yes to both questions, with some qualifying their answer to say the cesarean was definitely necessary for the baby's health. Overall, thirty-seven women answered yes to both questions, indicating that they trusted their doctor's decision and felt the cesarean was necessary. The other thirteen questioned the outcome to various degrees: four answered no to both questions; three answered no to 5, but yes to 6; three answered "not sure" to 5, but yes to 6; and three answered "not sure" to both 5 and 6.

All but one of the thirteen who questioned the cesarean decision later attempted a VBAC. In one way or another, most believed they could have delivered vaginally the first time if the doctor had done things differently or if they had had a different doctor. Joy of Alta, Wyoming had labored at home for sixteen hours and come to the hospital 8 centimeters dilated, when her doctor announced that something was "not quite right." He ordered an x-ray, which showed that the baby was in a breech position with his neck extended upward. He told the disappointed mother she would have to go to another hospital if she still wanted to attempt a vaginal delivery but that he was sure no one else would let her do it.

"Within 10 minutes, I had someone putting in a catheter, someone drawing my blood, and she couldn't find a vein in three attempts, and someone shaving my pubic hair and stomach," Joy wrote. "The doctor came in and yelled at the nurse who couldn't find the vein. All the while I was thinking 'this shouldn't be happening to me after my picture-perfect pregnancy.'" Though she ultimately believed the cesarean was necessary, Joy "felt a bit betrayed by the doctor because he didn't pick up on the fact that the baby was breech for so long." Just four days before her delivery, the doctor, who was known for his success at external cephalic version, had said the baby's position was fine. "I still don't think he was truthful," Joy wrote.

One other woman with a breech baby thought her doctor could have done more to promote a vaginal delivery. But the category of women who expressed the most skepticism about the need for their primary cesarean was the failure-to-progress group. Kendra of Richmond, Virginia wrote, "I felt that he gave up before I would have, but at the time I didn't feel I had any say in the decision. Nobody was in distress [though Kendra had stated that the baby had meconium, a possible sign of distress]; physically, everyone was fine."

Kathy of Virginia Beach wrote, "I asked the doc to let me labor a while longer [the baby's head was visible and Kathy had pushed for three hours], but he was concerned that the baby might go into distress. I wondered if the fact that both my husband and I are lawyers had anything to do with his decision. It was not an emergency when the cesarean was performed. On the other hand, I am grateful we had a healthy baby and that we did not get into a crisis situation." Kendra and Kathy each delivered two babies by VBAC.

Ellen of Houston also pushed for three hours. "The nurse asked him to let me keep trying," she wrote of her doctor. "He said I wouldn't do it and to set up the operating room after I'd only pushed a short time." She switched doctors and had a wonderful VBAC experience for baby number two.

Only one woman in the elective-cesarean group expressed uncertainty about whether her first cesarean was necessary. But there were two key differences between her story and those above. Jan of Algonquin, Illinois was so physically and emotionally traumatized by her labor and delivery experience that she was "terrified these things would happen again."

"These things" included a disagreement between the labor nurse (who thought she was 8 to 9 centimeters dilated) and a doctor (who thought she was "stuck" at 4 centimeters) when the doctor administered Pitocin. The nurse, whom Jan trusted more than the doctor, encouraged her to push when the doctor left the room. "Sometimes I think he went the other way because he didn't want her to contradict him and be right," she wrote. Jan also had complications from her epidural, which felt "great" until the anesthesiologist increased the medication for the surgery. She began shaking and vomiting (this is not uncommon), and eventually lost consciousness, which led to a five-hour stay in the recovery room.

"Whatever happened, I'm sure it wasn't supposed to, but I was at the mercy of those in control," Jan wrote. "I had *no* control at all at this point. It was a miserable experience. If I knew then what I knew the second time around, I really would have spoken up and questioned what was happening. Looking back, it was probably grounds for further examination legally."

Jan believes she was overdosed during the procedure and blames the medication, not the cesarean, on many of her problems recovering emotionally from the experience. None of the physical or emotional complications were recorded anywhere in her medical records. "We found it odd that these events were not important enough to document," she wrote. She waited five years to have another baby, and she found a doctor who was "understanding and eager to find out what had happened."

Jan was certain she wanted a repeat cesarean, and she also had a good medical reason: she was diagnosed with placenta previa early in the pregnancy, and the doctor could not tell for sure whether it had moved out of the way of the birth canal.

There was a qualitative difference between Jan's complaints and those of the women who wanted to attempt a VBAC. While the other women felt they could have lasted longer, endured more, pushed harder, Jan lost her sense of her physical ability to give birth in her first labor. She lost consciousness unexpectedly, a rather strong symbol of power loss. Furthermore, she unwillingly surrendered her control to a doctor she didn't trust. While the others came away from the first birth thinking "if only" they had had the chance, they could have pushed that baby out, Jan came away feeling disempowered, depressed, and robbed of self-confidence.

How Was the Baby at Birth?

Is there any connection between women's perceptions of their baby's health at birth and the method of delivery women preferred in the next pregnancy? Question 7 asked about the baby's condition at birth.

Forty of the fifty women answered "excellent," "healthy," "perfect," "fine," or "good" to the question about the baby's health, and many supplied Apgar scores.

Among the other ten women, Meg of Fort Worth, Texas had a baby who died sixteen hours after birth. He was born without a left lung and only part of the right lung. Meg subsequently gave birth to two healthy babies by elective repeat cesarean.

Nine other women expressed concerns of varying degrees about their baby's health. All nine either had a VBAC or attempted a VBAC in their next pregnancy. Three of the complaints came from women with breech babies. Patty of Spring, Texas had a baby with dislocated hips who was otherwise healthy. Joy said her baby's condition was "very good" but that he "had difficulty straightening out his legs" and "a very flat head" that was "always leaning over to the left." Joy said, "I have pictures of him with his feet up by his chin." Sarah of Virginia Beach complained that her baby's legs "stuck up for awhile due to his position in the womb." All of these positions are normal in breech babies.

Two babies spent time in intensive care, one because he was born six weeks premature (he's a tall, robust twelve-year-old now) and one who was healthy except for some respiratory problems. One woman's baby had a 1-minute Apgar score of 3 after swallowing blood from an abrupted placenta—his 5-minute score was 8. One baby had temporary breathing problems from inhaling meconium. And two mothers said their babies were blue at first, but then okay. None of the problems experienced by any of the babies were related to the cesarean birth.

Except for the mother whose baby died of congenital abnormalities, all thirteen of the mothers who opted for elective repeat cesarean in their next pregnancy reported their baby's condition as "perfect," "excellent," "normal," "fine," or "very good."

How Was Your Recovery?

Question 8 asked women whether they had any problems recovering from the cesarean and asked for the length of the hospital stay. This was meant to address physical recovery only, but some women wrote about emotional problems as well; those will be considered in the next section.

Interestingly, though the typical hospital stay for the cesarean women was the standard three to five days, there seems to be little correlation between the length of stay and the difficulty of recovery. In other words, some women who stayed only three days complained of tough recoveries, while some who stayed five or six reported no problems at all. This may be in part due to real differences in recovery times between one person and the next, to differences in policies about the timing of the discharge from the hospital, and to differences in the circumstances leading to the cesarean, such as the length of labor and the kind of anesthesia used. Specifically, four women who had general anesthesia complained a great deal about postoperative pain and difficulties nursing. Women whose surgery came on the heels of a long, hard labor complained about physical and mental exhaustion.

Forty-one of the fifty women said they did not have problems recovering from the cesarean. Of those, thirty opted for trial of labor in their next pregnancy, and eleven opted for repeat cesarean. Of the nine women who complained of difficult recoveries, seven opted for a trial of labor in the next pregnancy. Four of the nine had had general anesthesia for their primary cesarean.

One woman, Linda of Oak Park, Illinois, had a particularly disturbing experience in a Chicago hospital when she was twenty-one years old. Though the documented reasons for her cesarean were failure to progress and cephalopelvic disproportion, *she never felt any contractions* and was never told whether she had dilated. During a non-stress test on a Thursday afternoon, she was told she was in labor. She was given a sedative (Seconal) at the hospital, where she slept all night. She received general anesthesia for a cesarean at 10:30 the next morning. In short, she was completely drugged. Even worse, she was never informed of what was happening to her.

About her five-day hospital stay, Linda wrote, "It was horrible. The pain was terrible. I don't remember the first three days. I did develop an infection—a urinary tract infection, I think." After this experience, she trained to become a registered nurse and now works as an OB nurse. For her second pregnancy, she went to a midwife service at a Chicago teaching hospital and was vindicated by a very affirming and positive VBAC experience (see Chapter 8).

Martha of Chicago, who developed toxemia during her pregnancy in 1984, was in the pushing stage at the same Chicago teaching institution hospital when she told her attendants she felt pain between contractions. Alarmed by this complaint, and by the fact that her abdomen remained taut between contractions, they suspected a problem in her uterus, possibly an abrupting placenta. She underwent an emergency cesarean under general anesthesia and gave birth to a healthy baby boy of slightly low birthweight (5.5 lbs.).

"It took me over a year to feel the way I had felt before I was pregnant," she wrote. "It really hurt, I couldn't stand up or move easily for months. The incision seemed to take forever to heal, and when it did, it was an itchy red bumpy scar. I stayed in the hospital for eight days." She also lost her voice "from the tube they inserted when they put me under." Martha suffered another serious health problem, ulcerative colitis, during her second pregnancy three years later, and it wasn't accurately diagnosed until four months after the birth of her daughter, whom she delivered vaginally at the same hospital. Her second recovery also took a long time, due to the colitis, but she much preferred her VBAC.

Sue of Chicago had her cesarean in a suburban teaching hospital. She labored for three and a half days and only dilated to 3 centimeters. Her doctor had just examined her and was leaving, with his coat on, when the monitors suddenly indicated the baby was in distress. Sue had to have general anesthesia for an emergency cesarean. The baby had inhaled meconium and had initial respiratory difficulties. Sue reported problems finding a comfortable position for nursing and getting up from a supine position.

The fourth woman who underwent surgery with general anesthesia had her baby in a rural hospital. Lynette of Norfolk, Virginia, a registered nurse, came to the hospital fully dilated after only four hours of labor. She had some meconium-stained fluid. An ultrasound indicated the baby was a frank breech. Her doctor, who was at home in bed when Lynette arrived, came in and told her she would have to be sectioned. During *five* unsuccessful attempts to administer an epidural, the baby began to have decelerations and bradycardia, so Lynette had to have general anesthesia. The baby weighed only 5 pounds 2 ounces but had high Apgar scores.

"I had no epidural morphine and had a great deal of postoperative pain," Lynette complained of her five-day hospital stay. "I delivered at 8:20 A.M. and did not see my child until 6:30 P.M. I had an extremely hard time nursing my baby, and she only weighed 4 pounds 10 ounces when I left the hospital. I could not have my baby room in because she could not maintain her temperature." Lynette also complained of lack of assistance from her nurses.

For her next pregnancy, Lynette had a different doctor in the same medical practice; he pronounced her a good VBAC candidate but left the decision to her. "I had a hard time deciding," she wrote. "I knew I didn't want to repeat the first delivery scene." Her planned cesarean "went wonderfully (I was awake this time!)

and I had absolutely no discomfort. I went home on day two and had no trouble caring for a two-year-old and the new baby."

What all four women had in common is that none wanted to go through the same bad experience again. So why did Linda, Martha, and Sue opt for a trial of labor in their next pregnancy while Lynette opted for a repeat cesarean? Each of the women provides further clues about their decisions in their answers to subsequent questions. But every person experiences pregnancy and delivery with her own set of senses and unique responses, and giving birth *is* ultimately a matter of life or death. Nothing is more crucial in the mother's world at that moment. It's impossible to predict how a woman will sort through the wealth of data from the first birth to make the decisions that follow. What's important to recognize here is that each of the four women chose a different path the second time in order to improve upon her first experience, and in so doing, forged a much happier outcome. To rob women of these decision-making powers by persuading or requiring everyone to conform to one set of rules—a set of rules that may work for some but not others—is a violation of individual expression at one of life's most crucial moments.

Did You Feel Inadequate?

Asking women if they felt they had failed (question 9) was another attempt to differentiate between what women did and did not accept about their first experience. Did they internalize what happened as a negative reflection on themselves, something that they might have prevented if only they had been different? Or did they chalk it up to something over which they had no control, something that just happened but didn't reflect on them? Furthermore, did the surgery affect their ability to bond with the new baby?

As it turned out, there was substantial middle ground in the answers to this question. While five women, all of whom later wanted a VBAC, answered yes, they felt they had somehow failed, another fourteen women gave answers starting with "No, but . . . ," which typically contained the word "disappointed" or "discouraged" or "unhappy." Ten of these fourteen subsequently wanted a VBAC; four chose repeat cesarean.

Exploring first the women who felt they had failed, recall Sandra L., whose primary cesarean was done under a general anesthetic after an x-ray had showed her pelvis might be too small.

"Yes, I felt I had failed myself and my husband," wrote Sandra, who concealed her misery. "I was a child of the sixties and I always assumed that nature was the best choice. The intervention of surgery make me reexamine all sorts of conceptions I had about myself. If I were this very capable 'earth woman,' how could this have happened? Why couldn't I withstand the pain of labor? Was I just too old for motherhood? When I was pregnant for the second time I began reading tomes of material on VBAC and on unnecessary sections. I began to doubt my doctor and feel even more 'wimpy' than I had after the birth. There was nothing out there about women happy with themselves after a section. All the literature I found was geared toward a happy VBAC and an evil C-section. At best the C-section material was very clinical and never supportive of its positive benefits to mother and child or emotionally uplifting to those of us who have had them."

Sandra's self-image, like everyone's, was strongly influenced by the predominant culture around her. A cesarean delivery didn't mesh with the sixties, "earth woman" ideology she embraced. Interestingly, Sandra later acknowledged she was "quite certain the cesarean was necessary" and even recalled having an uncle who was severely retarded as a result of complications during his birth. Yet, for a short period of time, the negative cultural baggage associated with the surgery weighed more heavily on her than the positive medical reality, the medical blessing really, that enabled her baby and herself to survive childbirth unscathed.

Over time, Sandra's feelings about cesarean birth evolved, and she was able to own her positive feelings about the births of her other children despite what the books said she ought to be feeling.

The other women who felt they had failed—Martha and Sue, Alice of Tacoma, Washington, and Vicky of Ventura, California—

also complained of physical difficulties recovering or difficulties nursing.

"I felt my body had failed me, and I was angry for awhile that I didn't get to see my son being born," wrote Sue. "But those feelings passed and I started to appreciate that I had brought a precious new life home and that was more important—and I was still alive to be there for him and my family."

Vicky said her feeling of failure "faded away slowly." Alice said she was depressed and that the surgery had made breast-feeding difficult. Martha said she "was really depressed for almost the entire time I was in the hospital" (eight days), despite her doctor's efforts to cheer her up and explain why the cesarean had been necessary.

The fourteen women who answered "No, but..." didn't internalize their disappointment but tended to direct it outward—at the doctor, at the labor, at something about the situation.

Molly of Los Angeles said she felt, and still does feel, that perhaps other doctors would have tried harder for a vaginal delivery—she had pushed for three hours when her doctor advocated a cesarean—but she conceded she wasn't sure if "more trying would have been good" for the baby. Joy said she felt betrayed by her doctor because he "didn't pick up on the fact that my son was breech for so long." In other words, had the doctor picked up on it, they might have been able to turn the baby, and she might have delivered vaginally.

"I don't feel I failed, but I was certainly disappointed that I had to have a C-section," wrote Kendra, echoing a sentiment voiced by many of the women. "I had not anticipated it at all. I was in very good physical condition at the time of the birth. No one in my family had ever had one (Kendra has three sisters). I felt I had to do a lot of explaining to everyone about why I had a C-section." Not only did she feel she had to prove to herself she could deliver vaginally, she also felt she had to justify her cesarean to her family and friends. Kendra's older sister, who ended up with a cesarean with her first baby a short time later, felt similarly disappointed, and said she had done everything "by the book" in her pregnancy and hadn't expected or "deserved" that outcome.

Had something in their upbringing made them believe that real women don't have cesareans?

When planning for her VBAC, Kendra wrote, "I had convinced myself that it was a matter of strength and endurance that would or would not allow me to have a VBAC." Giving birth vaginally became a rite of passage for her, a notch of her true womanhood.

Conversely, giving birth vaginally carries no special meaning to other women. Shannon of Arlington Heights, Illinois said she had "a little" feeling of failure, which she got over by the third cesarean. "I think the failed syndrome is something people put in your head before the birth and make you believe," she wrote.

"I'm the type who does not particularly need the experience of a vaginal delivery to make my life whole!" wrote Talia of Glenview, Illinois. She and another mother wrote that women shouldn't feel guilty or that they had somehow failed by having a cesarean.

The question about bonding with their babies elicited an almost unanimous response of "no trouble bonding." A total of four women complained that bonding was difficult. All four said that bonding was delayed by either difficulties with breast-feeding or by the time required for the drugs to wear off (particularly with general anesthesia). One of the four, Lynette, also complained of lack of assistance from the nurses when she had difficulties breast-feeding her daughter, who weighed only 5 pounds. Of the four who reported delayed bonding, two preferred VBAC and two preferred repeat cesarean.

As might be expected, the women whose first cesarean did not sit well with them were more likely to want a VBAC in the subsequent pregnancy. And, in this particular group, the things that didn't sit well were not medical issues—none of the babies was harmed by surgery, and the women fared well physically for the most part—but what grated on them was their dashed expectations of a vaginal delivery. They knew what kind of delivery they had wanted, and the achievement of that goal had eluded them.

Conversely, the women who chose repeat cesarean did not seem particularly upset by the surgery but may have been emotionally traumatized by their labors. They also did not have serious complaints about their recoveries.

Women Who
Had VBACs

Twenty-six of the women who answered the surveys subsequently had a VBAC. In addition to the first nine questions about their cesarean birth (Chapter 7), they responded to ten questions about their VBAC experience.

Vaginal-Birth Questions

10. Same doctor or different one second time around? Hospital?

11. Choose one of the three to best describe your feelings about having a VBAC. a) I was certain I wanted to try a VBAC. b) I was certain I wanted to have an elective repeat. c) I was ambivalent and had a hard time deciding. Please explain reasons for your answer.

12. How did your doctor influence your decision? Did you at any time negotiate with your doctor? (for example, say you'd try a VBAC if your baby wasn't two weeks late and 9 lbs. like your first one; or you'd try a VBAC if you could have epidural anesthesia)

13. What actually happened? Did you go into labor on your own? Early, on time, or post due? Was labor induced for the VBAC?

14. Were drugs or other things (laminaria, prostaglandin)

used to induce or augment labor? How long was your labor?

15. Did you have an epidural or other painkilling medication? Were forceps or suction used? Did you have an episiotomy or tearing?

16. What was the baby's condition at birth? Was your bonding experience any different with this baby?

17. How did your recovery compare to the recovery from the C-section? Any problems resuming sexual intercourse? Any other problems? Hemorrhoids?

18. Overall, did you prefer one experience over the other? Why?

19. If you had another child, would you choose another VBAC?

Certainty or Ambivalence?

Of the twenty-six women who had a VBAC, twenty-three said they were certain they wanted to try a VBAC (choice a); the other three said they were ambivalent or had a hard time deciding (choice c).

The twenty-three women who expressed certainty about wanting to try VBAC gave an interesting variety of reasons. Eight women gave a medical reason. Four women gave the medical reason of wishing for a speedier recovery than they had had with their first cesarean, especially in light of already having another child at home to care for. Two women said they thought vaginal birth was a healthier option.

"I viewed the decision to have a C-section as stemming from circumstances that developed during the final stages of my pregnancy, i.e. our baby was breech, and not from any decision of mine or my doctor's to automatically have a C-section," wrote Karen of River Forest, Illinois. "Thus, in the absence of circumstances dictating the need for a C-section, I felt it was more appropriate, healthier, and preferable to have a vaginal delivery."

Only one woman, Jessica of Chicago, spoke directly about the issue of the safety of the incision. A nurse who had decided on her own she wanted a VBAC, Jessica said her doctor "did say the next one should be a VBAC—that the incision was such that it should not complicate a vaginal birth."

The last of the medical reasons came from Patty, who said, "I didn't want to compromise my abdominal wall anymore with another C-section."

Five women gave an "I can do it" reason for choosing to labor. One of the five, Mercedes of Ann Arbor, Michigan, had already experienced a vaginal delivery prior to her first cesarean, so she knew it was possible. Kendra wanted to prove to herself and perhaps others that she could do it. "I had convinced myself that it was a matter of strength and endurance that would or would not allow me to have a VBAC," she wrote. "I wanted the decision of 'going for it' to be mine." In her first pregnancy, her doctor had pulled the curtain on her labor at a point when she felt she could have continued.

Likewise, Kendra's friend Kathy looked at vaginal delivery as a challenge she could master. "Given the fact that I got to 7 centimeters unmedicated the first time with little pain, I knew I could do a vaginal delivery without an epidural, which had had a bad effect on my first labor." The baby's head had crowned in her first delivery, and she felt the epidural had prevented her from being able to push him out.

"Because I had known of many women who had had VBACs, I was sure I could have one," wrote Aleta of Chicago.

And Joy believed she could have delivered vaginally the first time if only her doctor had known the baby was breech and had tried to turn him. "The doctor's inattentive prenatal care was the reason my baby was in the wrong position for a vaginal delivery," she wrote. "At least if the breech position was unable to be corrected I would have been mentally prepared for its consequence. Physically, I should have had no problem."

Three women who were certain they wanted to try a VBAC said they wanted to know what it was like to "experience" vaginal birth.

"I wanted the experience," wrote Corrie of Alexandria, Virginia.

"I was told that the one good thing about my first ordeal [a ninety-hour labor with two hours of pushing] was that it would pave the way for success the second time," wrote Carla of Evanston, Illinois. "I did want to experience a vaginal birth."

And Daniela of Ann Arbor, Michigan said she felt "ripped off" by her scheduled cesarean for her first baby, who was breech. "I wanted to experience a vaginal birth as long as the baby was not at risk."

Two women indicated that they took their cue from doctors who advocated a VBAC. Moira of Chicago, who labored twenty-seven hours the first time and was dilated 4 centimeters when her placenta abrupted, wrote, "My doctor thought there was no reason why a vaginal birth would not be successful." And Amy of Santa Barbara said her doctor "strongly felt I should have a VBAC and I agreed easily."

One woman desperately wanted to avoid repeating her first experience, during which she was mostly unconscious. Linda never felt any contractions but was nevertheless drugged all night and sectioned under general anesthesia the following morning at a private hospital for failure to progress and cephalopelvic disproportion. "I had had a wonderful pregnancy only to be ruined by a dreadful, frightening birth and hospital experience," she wrote. "Going with the midwives [at a different, teaching hospital], I figured if I had even the slightest of chances for a VBAC, they were my best bet."

Four women who said they were certain they wanted to try VBAC didn't give reasons.

Of the remaining three VBAC women who were ambivalent, two had given birth to babies weighing 9 pounds or more the first time.

Kay, a Chicago physician, wrote, "I was ambivalent: It had been an intense labor and ultimately would probably not have been successful given the size of the baby [9 pounds, 8 ounces]. I saw no reason to think baby number two would be much smaller." She had dilated to 8 centimeters in eight hours in the first pregnancy but did not progress further. She developed a fever of 102 degrees, later found to be due to endometritis, and the baby was experiencing bradycardia.

The other woman with a 9-pound baby, Ellen, said she was certain his size was the reason she couldn't deliver him. "If the second baby was going to be large, I wanted another cesarean," she wrote. She had dilated fully and pushed for three hours before being sectioned.

Lastly, Jodi of Chicago had her first cesarean because the baby was breech, and an attempt to turn her hadn't worked. "I would have preferred another C-section, but I also wanted a different experience and to try a natural birth," she wrote. "Truthfully, though, I didn't feel like I had a choice; if the baby was in position, it was understood I would go with the vaginal birth." Her answer was truly ambivalent, to the point that she didn't or couldn't exercise a choice; the choice "was understood." This woman was one of three who, after having a VBAC, said she had preferred her cesarean delivery.

How Did Your Caregiver Influence Your Decision?

Most of the women, seventeen, said their doctor or midwife strongly supported and encouraged their desire to pursue a VBAC. These situations could be called "partnerships," in which the mother communicated her preferences early in the pregnancy, and the caregiver bolstered her choice.

One woman in this group, Kathy, a lawyer from Virginia Beach, wrote a birth plan for babies number two and three, which she said her doctor approved. (She stayed with the same physician group.) The birth plan, a copy of which she included with her survey, listed "vaginal delivery" as her goal and nine items as priorities. They were, as follows:

1. As much mobility as possible during all phases of labor.

2. Intermittent monitoring only as medically necessary. Pre-

fer no internal monitoring. Monitoring decisions to be discussed by doctor with patient.

3. No pain medication offered to patient. Allow patient to request if desired.

4. Allow patient to walk and/or shower during labor.

5. No IV until active labor is well established. IV decision to be discussed by doctor with patient.

6. Liberal time allowed for pushing.

7. Check dilatation before administering epidural.

8. Allow epidural to wear off somewhat during pushing.

9. No episiotomy if possible.

The birth plan "became standing orders of the doctor so when I went to the labor and delivery room, the nurses knew the agenda before the doctor arrived."

Another four women said their doctor "had no influence" in their decision or that "it was totally my decision." These situations could be called patient-directed, in which the mother attempted to control as much as she could, relying on the doctor mostly for technical expertise but not for advice or guidance. The remaining five women, conversely, indicated that their doctor told them a vaginal delivery would be expected and pursued; these situations could be called physician-directed.

Eighteen of the twenty-six women switched caregivers from their previous experience, either by choice or because of a move or an insurance change; only eight stayed with their first doctor or midwife.

One woman whose insurance had changed didn't like the doctor in her new health maintenance organization. "When I went to our new HMO's OB, he would only vaguely promise to attempt a VBAC," wrote Jessica. "It was also apparent that he had little experience with them. My running joke of him was that the only VBACs he was a party to were the ones that happened because he got to the hospital too late to do the C-section." Before she conceived the second time, she and her husband paid higher insurance premiums so that she could return to her first doctor. The change of insurance programs "guaranteed at least a shot at the VBAC."

One woman who apparently didn't have this degree of communication with her doctor ended up switching to someone else when she was eight and a half months pregnant. "I realized the doctor I had chosen was only going to let me labor two hours and preferred general anesthesia," wrote Natalie of Flossmoor, Illinois, whose plans for a home birth the first time around were dashed after thirty-six hours of labor. "I called a VBAC organization to get advice. I was given the name of a doctor who was known for letting women labor and deliver vaginally after C-sections." Natalie's demands may have exceeded those of other women. She didn't know her due date because she had become pregnant while nursing the first baby and didn't have menstrual periods. She wouldn't allow an ultrasound to determine the baby's gestational age, a decision which might have made many doctors refuse her case, especially at more than eight months into the pregnancy.

Four women were cared for by midwives in their subsequent pregnancy. One of the four, Carla, stayed with the same midwife group she had selected in her first pregnancy. "My midwife so strongly encouraged me to try VBAC that she made a personalized relaxation tape for me to use to prepare for 'opening up' in labor," wrote Carla. "I used it during pregnancy and fruitfully fell asleep almost every time. I did say that although I believed it was right to try a VBAC, I in no way wanted a repeat of my last experience and would cut the effort short if I felt things weren't going right. I also said if the baby was [occiput]posterior again, I would not try a VBAC." The other three women all sought out midwives because they said they wanted to maximize their chances of having a vaginal birth.

Perhaps the most important point to glean from these women's stories is the effort they expended to find a caregiver who supported their plans. Some women had to find a new caregiver and even change insurance policies to pursue their goal. Others were simply lucky in this regard. Karen said her Chicago doctor, the same one who had performed her cesarean for a breech presentation, initiated a discussion to ask the type of birth she envisioned next and said he would support her choice of a repeat section *or* a VBAC. When she asked what he recommended, he said he recommended she pursue whatever type of birth she wanted.

If only all women were so fortunate as to have a doctor like this! It's rare to find a doctor who is flexible enough to concede this much power to a patient. Some doctors may say the patient can choose what she wants but will still try to win her over to their agenda during the course of the pregnancy. (It's hard to fault them for that, as long as they are honest about their views and intentions.) It probably also helped Karen's cause to be well informed about her choices; otherwise her doctor might not have felt so comfortable letting her call the shots. Karen's story and the others illustrate the importance of good communication between mother and caregiver.

What Happened?

The simple answer is that all 26 women had a VBAC. Questions 13 through 15 asked for details such as whether the women went into labor on their own or had to be induced, how long they labored, whether Pitocin or epidurals were administered, and whether they had an episiotomy or forceps or vacuum suction.

Interestingly, all but two of the twenty-six women went into labor on their own; one was induced one and a half weeks past her due date, and the other at two weeks past. The shortest labor lasted just three and a half hours while the longest took four days. Daniela had contractions for four days that never got closer than five minutes apart. Upon entering the hospital she was given Pitocin, and the baby experienced heart-rate decelerations. But a scalp test (used to confirm the baby's oxygen level) confirmed that the baby was okay, and Daniela continued to labor, finally giving birth vaginally.

The average length of labor in this group was twenty-six hours (four women didn't include the length of time they labored). Only four women reported labors lasting less than ten hours. Given that the labors were relatively long, and that only six women reported having Pitocin to augment labor, it doesn't appear as if active management of labor was widely employed. The women either found caregivers who would let them labor indefinitely, or they labored at home for quite some time before coming to the hospital.

Seventeen women reported receiving epidural anesthesia. Nineteen said they had an episiotomy, and five said they had tears or lacerations (including one who had an episiotomy). Forceps or vacuum extraction were used in five of the deliveries.

Every woman has a unique story about each labor and delivery, and since these stories can't be quantified, what follows are several accounts of uplifting experiences, two accounts of experiences the women would rather not repeat, and one particularly unique account of a birthing position advocated by a midwife.

First, the positive experiences. For her first delivery, Linda had been put to sleep overnight at a Chicago hospital and then sectioned the next morning under general anesthesia. The documented reasons for her cesarean were failure to progress and cephalopelvic disproportion, but she had never felt a contraction and was never told whether she had dilated. During her second pregnancy, Linda used the midwife service at a university teaching hospital in Chicago. She went into labor three days past her due date and stayed at home all day until she could no longer talk through her contractions. Her daughter was born three and a half hours after she arrived at the hospital. She received one dose of a painkiller and had no episiotomy, but she did have a second-degree laceration.

"Our daughter was fine," she wrote. "The whole experience was wonderful. My husband was there this time and could participate. I was awake and aware. I remember everything this time. It was as if I had scripted it. She went to breast immediately—I could go on and on."

Several other women wrote of relatively short labors with no need for interventions. Though Aleta didn't say how long she labored, she too had an upbeat experience. "I began labor on my own on my due date," she wrote. "At the hospital, I refused to have my bag of waters ruptured, and I insisted on being sent home until it was absolutely necessary to be in the hospital. When I arrived at the hospital, I was fully dilated. Then I delivered vaginally without problems."

Kathy enjoyed her first VBAC. She went into labor one week past her due date and stayed at home with "easy cramps" for fifteen hours. Arriving at the hospital when her contractions were five minutes apart, she delivered three hours later. "No internal monitoring, no Pitocin, no epidural or any pain medications, no forceps or vacuum, no episiotomy, minor lacerations," she wrote. "I squatted to push and the baby came out after three pushes." Kathy had another VBAC with a third child, as did five other women in this group. Though she broke her coccyx (tail bone) while squatting to push out baby number three, she nonetheless reported feeling good enough that she could have gone back to work the following day. The other five women all said their second VBAC was easier than the first, as is typical for any subsequent vaginal delivery.

"My husband and I have a third child," wrote Karen. "He was born by VBAC in the type of comfortable, warm and fuzzy birth that everyone should have at least once."

Two women had complained about exceptionally traumatic cesarean experiences and had equally bad VBAC experiences. Joy had been angered by her first cesarean because she felt that the doctor, an expert at external cephalic version, should have known (or did know) that her baby was breech long before the delivery, but didn't diagnose it with an x-ray until she was 8 centimeters dilated, at which point she was rushed into surgery.

For her second delivery, Joy labored at home for eleven hours and came to the hospital 5 centimeters dilated. Then she labored another sixteen hours at the hospital. "There was suction, and forceps, and an episiotomy clear down to my knee (clearly an exaggeration but a huge episiotomy in any case), used at the end," she wrote, explaining that the size of the episiotomy represented a desperate attempt to get the baby out. "The fetal monitor had come off and when they replaced it and found that the baby was not doing well, the doctor delivered the baby in about one minute. He was in a panic and clearly concerned for the baby." The baby sustained head injuries, wasn't breathing, and was taken away for ten minutes. "The next morning when the doctor made his rounds he commented that he thought he had killed my baby." She did not appreciate this remark. The baby did not calm down for twelve hours, but was eventually okay. Joy still had not fully recovered from the physical effects of the birth three years later.

Carla had labored ninety hours (eighty-four hours at home) and pushed for two hours before her first cesarean was done for failure to descend. She used a midwife up until the time of the cesarean. In retrospect, she felt the cesarean should have been done sooner, "for my sake, because I was so wiped out from no sleep and then also had to recover from surgery."

In the second pregnancy, Carla's water broke a week early, a short time after an internal exam "at which I think some help was given, on the assumption that an earlier baby would be easier for me." She said she had a smallish pelvic opening but really did want to experience a vaginal birth, and her midwife had prepared a special relaxation tape for her.

Her contractions, like the first time, were widely spaced and unproductive. She was admitted to the hospital at 9 A.M., five hours after her water broke, and then given Pitocin. She was "in dire misery by noon and begging for relief," she wrote. "Got epidural shortly after (to the disgust of my midwife, who said, 'Well, you can't walk around anymore now!')"

Unfortunately, the epidural didn't work properly and "seemed only to shift the pain from center to left—no pain reduction. I asked for and got more; no change. I began begging for a C-section. If it had occurred to me, I would have asked to be put out completely; fortunately, I forgot it was an option. Labor was sixteen hours, eight of which were hideous." She, too, has had significant physical problems since the VBAC.

"A major disappointment to me in the VBAC was the feeling that my midwife—even my husband, but briefly—discouraged the epidural and wanted me to just 'relax' instead. I felt they had *no idea* what I was feeling and didn't trust me to know."

One woman had a unique experience with a midwife. Melanie of Danville, California wanted to do everything possible to have a VBAC—she had her cesarean because of twins—so she, too, switched from a doctor to a midwife. It took only seven hours of labor before she was fully dilated, at 6 A.M.

"That's when the problems started," she wrote. "The baby was big and he was at 0 station and wouldn't progress. I pushed and pushed without results. The midwife had been with me since about 4:30 A.M. and tried having me squat, sit on the toilet, etc., with no results. The contractions continued to be horrendous so I decided I needed an epidural. They gave me just enough epidural to take the edge off but not enough to inhibit the pushing. Still, the pushing was doing nothing and the midwife wasn't sure what to do. Fortunately, her shift was over at 8 A.M. and the new midwife who relieved her knew exactly what to do. She put me in *trendelenburg* (head down, feet up) and had me push. She guided me constantly, putting her fingers on my perineum with each contraction to give me direction in which to push. It was slow but the baby started to make movement. In all I pushed for four hours but managed to be successful with a vaginal birth."

Though a doctor was available in the event Melanie needed a cesarean, she believes there's no question she would have ended up with another cesarean with a physician as her primary attendant. The baby had high Apgars, 8 and 9, and weighed 9 pounds 4 ounces. Melanie said she had a harder time recovering from the VBAC because she developed an infection postdelivery that made it painful to walk. She thought the infection may have been caused by the midwife's hands on her perineum.

Some of the women were fortunate to have relatively easy vaginal deliveries. Others had difficult vaginal deliveries. The women who didn't seem to mind the difficult deliveries were the ones who were most committed to VBAC at the outset.

How Was the Baby at Birth?

Five women of the twenty-six reported problems with the baby at birth, while the other twenty-one said the baby was "excellent," "healthy," "fine," or "perfect." One baby was born with a temporary blood sugar problem (likely having nothing to do with the mode of delivery). Another was born with torticollis, a condition in which the neck muscles on one side are in spasm, causing the head to pull over to one side. The mother does not know the origin of the baby's problems but suspects they might be congenital. The baby received physical therapy and is now fine.

Three other babies were not breathing at birth. One mother did not provide details except to say her baby was stressed, lacked oxygen, and was taken away at birth. He is fine now. Stacy of Ojai, California wrote, "Due to cord wrapped around neck and speed of delivery, the baby was not breathing; needed intubation; scary." He is also fine.

Lastly, Joy, whose baby was delivered by a doctor "in a panic" after the fetal monitor came off and the baby was found to be in distress, wrote, "the baby's condition was not good. The staff basically left me for about ten minutes and worked on the baby. He was not breathing and had head injuries from the suction and forceps, and a huge bump on his forehead where he had been pounded by my pelvic bone. He was very blue for a long time. He didn't calm down for at least twelve hours. It was very difficult." This baby was also okay. But the problems he suffered, and those of the other resuscitated babies, are much more common in vaginal deliveries than in cesarean deliveries.

Most of the women said bonding with their baby was the same or a little easier. Stacy and Joy said they had more trouble, as did two other women who said they were simply too exhausted after their birth ordeal to bond well. "I had more trouble bonding because I felt so bad after the birth," said Natalie of Flossmoor, Illinois. And Jodi of Chicago, who had been ambivalent about attempting a VBAC, said, "After two and a half hours of pushing, I was more relieved that he was out of me than that he was here." Jodi labored for two and a half days before the birth.

How Was Your Recovery?

Considering that one of the selling points of VBAC is easier recovery, it was somewhat surprising that only fourteen of the twenty-six women, just over half, said their recovery was easier. Five said recovery from VBAC was more difficult, and another seven gave mixed reviews. Those who said the recovery was harder complained of lacerations (fourth degree in one case), severe hemorrhoids, significant discomfort from the episiotomy, and painful sexual intercourse. Carla said she still had discomfort sitting down a year after the birth and "sex hurt way more than before."

Among the mixed reviews was that of Daniela, the mother who labored for four and a half days and who was cared for by a staff of midwives (plus her best friend, who is also a midwife). "I could walk around and get in and out of bed easier," she wrote, four months after the birth. "However, my bottom was very sore. I still fear pain with intercourse." At the urging of her friend, she left the hospital early to recover at home, only to have to return two nights later with a fever of 102 degrees and a uterine infection. In addition, she had a bladder problem, and her bilateral labial tears, which had required six stitches, still hadn't healed one week postpartum. Her caregiver instructed her to take four sitz baths a day, to which Daniela responded, "How I am going to find time for that?" Nonetheless, she thought recovery might have been worse with a cesarean.

Another mixed review came from Karen. "The VBAC recovery was quicker than that of the C-section in that I did not have any of the abdominal discomfort associated with the C-section," she wrote. "Conversely, my hemorrhoids were so unbearable that I barely had a chance to react to the discomfort of the episiotomy, which wasn't insignificant. Sexual intercourse resumed, as evidenced by our third child, but I don't recall it being all fun and games at first, regardless of my husband's attempts to make it so."

And Kay, the Chicago physician, reported a more difficult recovery with the VBAC. "The hemorrhoids of the VBAC were worse than the section surgical wound!" she wrote. "I felt like bronzing that first BM! It was difficult to stand up for more than a few minutes at a time for several weeks. No special problems with intercourse (when we were finally awake enough to go for it)."

The most sobering and serious report of post-VBAC suffering came from Joy. "I am still recovering from the last birth," she wrote, three years after the VBAC birth. "I do at least a hundred kegels a day and am still having a bladder control problem stemming from the stretching out and non-elasticity of my vaginal wall, or at least that is what my current doctor is saying is the root of this problem. I can still feel where the episiotomy is and at times have aches there. For months I suffered with pain from that incision and felt an actual loss of my walking ability for the first few weeks. My rectum is still misshapen and actually pooches out from the force of that birth. Intercourse has never been the same. The loss of muscle tone makes it difficult."

Most women do not have such serious complications after a vaginal delivery. But among the twenty-six VBAC women, there were twelve complaints about hemorrhoids and twelve relating to episiotomies, tears, or painful sexual intercourse. Joy's symptoms are more typical of someone who has had multiple vaginal deliveries. Injuries incurred to the female genital and anal areas, injuries that may affect female sexual response, tend to be downplayed by an obstetrical community largely dominated by males. And women may also underreport such problems because they aren't easy to talk about—divulging details about the quality of one's sex life is still somewhat taboo in our society. Furthermore, perhaps women feel, as many expressed in their surveys, that since vaginal birth is nature's intended mode of delivery, it isn't right to complain about the complications that accompany it.

Some experts argue that nature did not endow humans with an exceptionally good mode of birth. "As an obstetrician, as chairman of my department for the last twenty years, I came to the conclusion that vaginal delivery is not the best kind of delivery," says M. Maurice Abitbol, M.D., of the Jamaica Hospital in Jamaica, New York. "We have a mode of birth which is not the best in the universe. Nature didn't do perfectly well in this matter."

Furthermore, he says, "The sexual life of women who have an elective cesarean section is much better than of those who have a vaginal delivery, no question about it." The reason, he says, is that vaginal delivery can adversely affect the birth canal, the perineum, and the vaginal structure.

For some women, such difficulties may never occur; for others, they resolve in time. Where the majority of women would fall on the spectrum of sexual difficulties following vaginal childbirth is anyone's guess, since it's not a subject that has been widely investigated or even discussed. But an obstetrician who speaks in favor of cesarean section has little or nothing to gain these days, so Dr. Abitbol's statements may be worth consideration, at the very least by an individual in the position of choosing the mode of delivery she prefers.

Which Experience Did you Prefer?

The final questions on the VBAC survey, 18 and 19, asked women which experience they preferred and why, and whether they would choose VBAC again if they had another child. Most of the women, seventeen of twenty-six, said they preferred the vaginal delivery. The reasons they gave included easier recovery; "that's how it was meant to be"; that the delivery was more exciting; that both parents were more involved; that there was more of a victorious feeling; and that the mother could see the baby being born.

Six women said they didn't prefer one method over the other or couldn't decide.

"It was nice to have had a vaginal birth given that I'd had a C-section the first time," wrote Karen. "However, 'experientially,' it might also be nice to go through Army boot camp as a means of initiating an exercise regimen, but one might not always make that choice again. In retrospect, I never thought a C-section was that bad ... there was more abdominal discomfort, but in my case, at least, it meant that labor was over fast, the baby and I were okay, and I never perceived that I had somehow 'failed.'

However, as one still living with the hemorrhoidal effects of a long push [in her first VBAC], I wasn't all too thrilled about that aspect of the recovery. Moreover, following that delivery, I definitely believe that labor was called labor for a reason...by the forty-eighth hour, it was no longer a dewy-eyed, warm and fuzzy experience. So, all in all, it's a toss-up in my book." As mentioned earlier, Karen's third delivery was the charm.

The other three women said they preferred the cesarean. "It was relaxed, quicker, cleaner, and less painful," said Jodi about her cesarean, sans labor, for breech presentation. Joy also preferred her cesarean, as did Kay, the Chicago physician.

As for what they would do next if the occasion presented itself, twenty-one of the twenty-six women said they would choose another VBAC, four said they would choose cesarean, and one gave a mixed response. Despite some negative consequences of vaginal birth, most notably the recovery problems experienced by Joy, and, to a lesser extent, a few other women, the vast majority of the twenty-six women had positive experiences.

Some questions to ponder if you are interested in VBAC: To what lengths are you willing to go to have a VBAC? How long are you willing to labor? And what interventions are you willing to accept or not accept?

Women Who
Wanted VBACs

There were twelve women in the group of fifty who wanted to deliver vaginally but ended up with a repeat cesarean. Ten of the twelve labored before they were sectioned; the other two wanted to labor and had doctors who were amenable, but medical circumstances near the time of birth dictated a cesarean. Following are the questions they answered about their attempted or intended vaginal delivery.

Repeat-Cesarean Questions

10. Your age when you had repeat cesarean. Same doctor or different one second time around? Same or different hospital?

11. Choose one of the following to best describe your feelings about having a cesarean again. (a) I was certain I wanted to try a VBAC and did. (b) I wanted to try a VBAC but my doctor wouldn't go along with it. (c) I was certain I wanted to have an elective repeat cesarean because . . . please explain. (d) I was ambivalent and had a hard time deciding. Please elaborate on any of these answers if you'd like.

12. How did your doctor influence your decision? Did you at any time negotiate with your doctor? (For example, say

you'd try a VBAC if your baby wasn't two weeks late and 9 lbs. like your first one, or you'd try a VBAC if you could have epidural anesthesia?)

13. What actually happened? Did you have an elective repeat cesarean, did you try to have a VBAC, or did something else occur?

14. What was the baby's condition at birth?

15. How long did you stay in the hospital? Any trouble bonding with the baby?

16. How did your recovery compare to the recovery from your first cesarean? Any complications?

17. Was the second cesarean easier or harder overall than the first one?

18. If you had it to do over again, which birth option would you choose, cesarean or vaginal birth?

Certainty or Ambivalence?

This group of twelve women was as determined to pursue VBAC as the group in Chapter 8 who succeeded. In response to question 10, ten of the twelve women indicated they were certain they wanted to try a VBAC (choice a).

One woman, Cindy of Westport, Connecticut gave an equivocal answer but did want to try VBAC. She wrote, "I was ambivalent but didn't have a hard time deciding. I was nervous about having a VBAC, just because I hadn't had a vaginal delivery the first time, so I wasn't sure what to expect, but felt that if I could have a vaginal delivery, I wanted to try to do it that way."

The twelfth woman, June of Chicago, indicated she was ambivalent and had a hard time deciding (choice d). Her first baby had been a footling breech, and she had been sectioned without laboring. She wasn't all that eager to labor in her second pregnancy. "I wasn't sure that I wanted to experience labor and actually wanted to have an elective C-section," she wrote. "My doctor pushed for a VBAC because she said my recovery would be shorter and it would be easier with my seventeen-month-old son. I wasn't completely convinced that I wanted a VBAC, but my doctor's reasoning made sense, so I went along with a VBAC."

How Did Your Caregiver Influence Your Decision?

Eight of the twelve women said their doctors "supported," "encouraged," or "agreed with" their desire to pursue a VBAC. As in Chapter 8, these relationships could be termed partnerships. Sonia of Dayton, Ohio seemed to have a communicative partnership with her second doctor, a woman at a military hospital. Sonia's first cesarean had been performed for fetal distress after she had labored for twenty-four hours and dilated to 8 centimeters. "My doctor advocated VBAC because with C-section, there is a longer recovery time and always a chance of infection," she wrote. "She told me it was my decision, however." At 40 weeks' gestation, after performing an ultrasound and estimating the baby's size at 8 pounds, her doctor asked her if she would like to be induced to increase her chances of having a successful VBAC.

By contrast, two women reported that their doctors essentially made the decision for them to pursue a VBAC. These were physician-directed situations. In the case of Amy of Santa Barbara, her doctor's assumption that she would have a VBAC ("C-section wasn't considered," she wrote) was bolstered by the fact that her second baby had been delivered vaginally, following her first baby's birth by cesarean. Moreover, Amy agreed with the doctor's assessment, as the second birth had gone well. June said her doctor "really wanted to try for a VBAC," even though June "actually wanted to have an elective C-section." June and her doctor "did agree that if I went into labor and didn't progress over a reasonable period of time that we would go ahead with a C-section."

The other two women made their decision known to their physician—their choice was patient-directed. Julia of Los Angeles said, "My doctors always did what I told them I wanted to do." And Cindy wrote, "My doctor did little to influence my decision other than to say it was okay to try a VBAC."

None of the twelve women in this group went to a midwife. Nine went to a different doctor in their second pregnancy.

What Happened?

The women's answers to question 13 reveal what actually happened during the trial of labor and why they ended up having a cesarean.

As noted previously, two of the women, Vicky of Ventura, California, and Sandra of Oshkosh, Wisconsin, were sectioned before labor. Sandra followed her doctor's advice to have a cesarean one week after her due date had passed. She had a small pelvic opening and, in addition to being late, the second baby was estimated to be bigger than the first. Moreover, Sandra wanted to be awake during the delivery, and at her hospital, a spinal or epidural would be used for an elective surgery but should a cesarean become necessary during labor, general anesthesia would be used. This policy further discouraged her from pursuing a trial of labor. After the first cesarean baby, Sandra had three more children by repeat cesarean, all at the same hospital and with the same doctor.

Vicky's doctors recommended a cesarean after a series of ultrasounds and non-stress tests beginning a month before her due date indicated that she had too much amniotic fluid. On a Friday, a few days before her due date, they told her the baby was full term and "wanted out." Vicky suggested she would go home and think about it, but the doctors said they wanted her to stay on the monitor in the hospital.

Vicky so wanted a vaginal delivery that she had hired a labor coach. She called the labor coach, who questioned why the doctors wouldn't consider an induction. "This was never an option," Vicky wrote. "They didn't feel it would be good for the baby to be delivered vaginally." Though she was very upset, the monitor was showing that the baby was in distress, so she agreed to a cesarean that afternoon.

"All I could do was trust what my doctors were saying," she wrote. "My attention was turned away from my desire to deliver vaginally and towards the health of my baby and myself. I knew from experience that everything would be okay, since I had been down this road before. I agreed to the cesarean and felt good about my decision." The baby girl had the umbilical cord wrapped around her neck three times, but her condition after surgery was fine.

Though she accepted the fact that the surgery was medically indicated, Vicky did not like the way her doctor had communicated with her. On one occasion he addressed her husband as if Vicky weren't there. "My husband was with me, and the doctor said to him, 'If it were my wife I would want her to have a C-section.'" Adults may make such decisions for their children, but not for their spouses, unless the person is mentally incompetent. Vicky resented being treated so insensitively. As she was very committed to VBAC and driven to tears when she learned it wasn't feasible, she should have received extra empathy and patience from her caregivers. Instead, her feelings were dismissed. It would have been more appropriate for the doctor to have spoken to Vicky directly: "If you were my wife or my sister, I would want you to have a C-section."

Vicky suspected there was an additional motive to perform a cesarean. Her baby was due December 21, and the doctor had said that she could "have this baby by noon, well before Christmas." While Vicky may have received adequate medical care, she had little or none of the emotional support that a VBAC candidate in particular sometimes needs.

The other ten women in the group went through labor. One woman had a cesarean after her baby, which had been head-down a week earlier, was discovered to be breech during labor (her first cesarean was also done for breech presentation). The other nine women ended up with a cesarean for failure to progress or failure to descend, including at least four who had dilated fully and pushed. Among the nine with failure to progress or descend, five had had their first cesarean for fetal distress, two for failure to progress, and two for breech presentation. It is hard to draw any conclusions from this small group about any relationship between the medical reasons for the first and second cesareans. But what does seem apparent is that failure to progress or failure to descend, sometimes touted as a weak reason for cesareans, is in fact often what happens. These are true cases of "the baby won't come out."

What was also noteworthy about three of the women who dilated fully and pushed was that all had babies in the occiputposterior position (the back of their heads were hitting the back of the mother's pelvis). Babies in this position have more difficulty passing successfully through the birth canal, according to Gary Thurnau, M.D., the investigator of the fetal-pelvic index (see Chapter 3, page 39). Sometimes these babies can be turned manually; other times they cannot.

June, whose doctor wanted the VBAC more than she did, labored for fifteen hours, including two and a half hours of pushing, only to end up with a repeat cesarean. "The baby was facing upwards, and he was wedged in and wasn't coming out," she wrote. "My doctor tried to move him while I was pushing, but he would not move. So, after all the labor, I ended up having a C-section." Recall that June's doctor had agreed to perform a C-section if she didn't progress over a "reasonable" period of time. Two and a half hours of pushing was not June's understanding of reasonable.

Amy and Sonia had similar stories. Both had had their first cesarean for fetal distress and were nine days past due with the second baby when they were induced. Sonia had a device called a foley bulb inserted to induce labor. She was sent home and told that the bulb would fall out when she was 3 to 4 centimeters dilated. Her contractions started immediately and grew very intense. "But the bulb never fell out, so I remained at home until the pain was too unbearable," she wrote. "When I got to the hospital, I was 9 centimeters! Of course, mine was the first foley bulb to malfunction! Needless to say, I was unable to receive an epidural."

Sonia pushed for three and a half hours while her doctor tried unsuccessfully to turn the baby, who was occiputposterior. The doctor also tried suction. After this too failed, "My doctor mentioned C-section as an option," Sonia wrote. She pushed a while longer, then agreed. "I was exhausted and wanted to see my baby! Because I had had a previous C-section, the thought of one did not scare me."

Amy's experience was very similar except she was induced with Pitocin and also given an epidural. However, the epidural didn't work well, and she dilated to 10 centimeters in two hours, with back labor. Suction was applied three times, but the baby's heart rate decelerated significantly each time and the head would not budge. When the doctor became worried about how the baby would fare coming down the birth canal, he "strongly recommended a C-section, and we rapidly agreed," Amy wrote.

One woman, Julia, had her first and second cesareans for failure to descend. Though her twelve-hour second labor was fourteen hours shorter than the first, both times she pushed for about an hour, and the baby wouldn't come out. The second time, however, she wrote, "I began feeling like my previous scar was tearing and I was scared to keep trying. I was fully dilated, but the baby hadn't moved past zero position, so I had an epidural and another C-section." When she had her third baby, by elective cesarean, her doctor said her uterus was "paper thin" and would have ruptured had she gone into labor.

The other women in the failure-to-progress category labored between twelve and thirty-six hours before they gave birth by cesarean. One woman, Nora of Poway, California, had labored thirty-two hours the first time and only dilated to 2 centimeters; the second time she labored thirty-six hours and again only dilated to 2 centimeters. "The doctor said it was my decision, and I chose the C-section with spinal anesthesia rather than be there any longer."

How Was the Baby at Birth?

Most of the women who ended up with a cesarean reported that their baby's condition was "good," "very good," "excellent," or "healthy." Only two of the twelve women answered differently.

Amy, who was induced and dilated fully before the cesarean was performed for failure to descend, reported her baby's condition as "okay." His Apgar scores were 4 and 7, and the umbilical cord was wrapped around his neck, but he was fine within five minutes.

Sue of Chicago had her second baby at a university teaching hospital that happens to be very pro-VBAC. She didn't go into labor on her own and was finally induced two weeks past her due date. An ultrasound estimated the baby's size at 9 pounds (her first son had weighed 9 pounds 13 ounces). Sue labored for more than twenty-eight hours after the induction, including fifteen hours after her water had broken. She was examined frequently and developed an intrauterine infection over the course of the long labor. Finally, the doctors, who had "wanted to do the cesarean much earlier," insisted on it. Her baby, who had excreted meconium in utero and had to be "watched very closely for twenty-four hours," weighed *11 pounds 12 ounces*. (Sue did not have gestational diabetes, which can lead to excessive fetal growth.) Ultrasound images have a high rate of error when the baby is very small or very large, and Sue's experience points to the need for more accurate ways to estimate fetal size. Though her doctors may have let her labor longer than was probably wise, both for her sake and the baby's, Sue was satisfied with the outcome because she had done everything she could to strive for a vaginal delivery. Of course, she says now, had she known he was so big, she never would have attempted a VBAC.

Sue was the only mother who reported having bonding troubles with her baby. "The bonding process with him was much different," she wrote. "I didn't nurse with him as frequently due to the bottle feedings the nurses were giving him. Because he was such a big baby, the pediatrician wanted to make sure he got his nutrients every three to four hours. So by the time he would be brought to me, he would fall asleep after the first five minutes of breastfeeding. I really felt like the bonding process in that way was sabotaged."

How Was Your Recovery?

Questions 16 and 17 asked about the recovery process, the length of the hospital stay, and whether this recovery was easier or harder than the one following the first cesarean.

Seven of the twelve women reported an easier recovery, three said recovery was similar, and two said it was more difficult.

Counted among the seven who reported an easier recovery were the two women, Vicky and Sandra, who had had their cesareans without going through labor. Several others said having a shorter labor made their recuperation period shorter and easier.

"I recovered quickly from the incision," Vicky wrote. "I did not have postpartum depression and it seems my recovery was much quicker. I think it's because I didn't go through seventeen hours of labor before the operation. Also, I knew what to do and what to expect. The experience helped."

Sandra was even more upbeat. "I felt great," she wrote. "I used a morphine drip that did cause itching but easily covered my pain; in fact I felt as euphoric as that drug can make one feel. I never felt ill in any way, nor did I get the rumored spinal headache. The numbness lasted two hours at most." She also said the second birth was easier psychologically. "The only hard part was giving up the baggage of trying to have a VBAC that, I once felt, would assure my womanhood. "Once I let go of that concept, I was completely joyous. All the material I had read about the terrific VBAC really worked against me—against my psyche. I wish I had had an uplifting source of literature on a spiritual experience with another C-section to support me, rather than the *Silent Knife* sentiments I'd drenched myself in."

One woman who said her recovery was easier, Cindy, worked in her garden the day she returned home from the hospital, after a four-day stay. Even though the second labor was harder, she said the experience overall was easier "because we didn't wait so long to do it."

Two women who had anticipated a more difficult recovery the second time said they actually recovered more easily. Sonia did not labor as long in her second pregnancy but pushed for three hours before having a cesarean. "For some reason, after just a few hours' sleep, I felt totally rejuvenated," she wrote. "I was very surprised at how much more quickly I recovered from my second C-section. I was up and walking around (slowly!) twenty-four hours after surgery. I felt back to normal after only ten days—a little sore, but good."

June said she also recovered more easily from her second cesarean, even though she labored and pushed for two and a half hours the second time, and hadn't labored at all the first time due to the footling-breech presentation of the baby. Though she said she was extremely tired the first day after surgery and had a bad reaction to some pain medication, June felt fine thereafter and left the hospital in three days. She speculated that the recovery may have proceeded more smoothly because she knew what to expect.

Of the two women who said recovery was harder, Sasha of Chicago, said she was not as fit when she became pregnant the second time and didn't walk as soon after the second delivery. "I had more help, yet didn't seem to heal as quickly," she wrote. She labored twelve hours in the second pregnancy, six in the first.

Nora said her recovery was more difficult, even though she didn't have complications. "I labored longer and with no epidural and was more tired," she wrote. Also, her insurance covered only two days in the hospital, a deplorable trend that puts both mothers and babies at greater risk for developing complications that may not be readily identifiable. While several states have passed laws prohibiting insurance companies from instituting "drive through" delivery policies, further vigilance and political measures are needed to stop this trend.

What Would You Do If You Had Another Baby?

Question 18 asked women which birth option they would choose if they were having another baby, a cesarean or an attempted VBAC. Six women said they would have an elective cesarean, five said they would try for VBAC, and one gave an unclear answer.

Among the six who would choose an elective cesarean, three actually did have another child or two.

"I felt after two tries at a vaginal birth, there was no point in going through labor when I would be likely to end up with another C-section," wrote Charlene, who had her third baby via elective cesarean. "A positive point: I never had to have an episiotomy."

Sandra, who had two more elective cesareans to complete her family of four children, wrote, "For fleeting moments during each pregnancy, I longed to have a vaginal delivery, but I did not pursue it. The joy of being aware of my second child's birth was all I needed. At forty [her age when her third child was born], I knew that my bones didn't want to adjust themselves for an 8-pound-plus package sliding through, either."

June, who pushed for two and a half hours before being sectioned the second time, said not only would she choose cesarean if she had another child but that she wished she had stood firm on her desire to have one with baby number two. Rather than blaming her doctor, however, she faulted herself for being talked into a trial of labor she never wanted. She did indicate, however, that she would look for a different doctor if she became pregnant again.

Cindy explained her choice by saying that although both of her C-sections were uneventful, neither was elective: "I did have to go through full labor both times first."

The five women who said they would try VBAC again included Amy, who had already had one VBAC before having a cesarean with her third baby. Her reason: "Only because recovery is so much shorter and risks at birth are lower *if all goes well*."

Sonia, who, like Amy, went through complete labor before experiencing failure to descend, said she too would opt for VBAC but did not say why: "If I had to have a C-section, I would not be upset, because the end product is the same, hopefully—a healthy baby!"

Amy said she didn't mind her cesareans but would still try VBAC again if she had another baby.

Vicky said she would look harder for a doctor who would do everything possible to deliver the baby by VBAC. "I might look into a birthing center," she wrote. "But I would be the first to agree to a C-section if that doctor recommended it. At my age and with my history I would not want to take any chances." (Vicky was forty-one when her second baby was born.)

· · ·

In summary, only two women of the twelve, Vicky and June, seemed significantly disappointed by their second experience. What disturbed Vicky wasn't the cesarean itself—she felt physically and emotionally better about it than her first cesarean— but the callous way she was treated by her doctor and his partners. And what bothered June was that she was persuaded to do something she did not particularly want; having it not work was what she had wanted most to avoid.

The most likely explanation for the general acceptance of the outcomes by the rest of the group is that they had tempered their expectations of a vaginal delivery. They wanted a VBAC but had given serious thought about the possibility of ending up with another cesarean; several said they did not fear that outcome because they knew what to expect. Also, they did not put too much of themselves or their egos at stake when they attempted a trial of labor, so they didn't feel like failures when it didn't work.

This group of women came across as stable, optimistic, and very accepting of what had happened. The fact that several women expressed a willingness to go a third round with a trial of labor after it had twice failed further points to their lack of fear and to their acceptance of either outcome.

Women Who Had Elective Cesareans

There were a total of 16 women in the group of 50 who chose to have a repeat cesarean. Thirteen women opted for the surgery in the pregnancy immediately following their first delivery. The other three, Julia of Los Angeles, Charlene of Montclair, New Jersey, and Sandra of Oshkosh, Wisconsin had an elective repeat with their third child after a VBAC attempt in the second pregnancy (or a desire to attempt VBAC, in Sandra's case) did not work out. Sandra also had a fourth cesarean.

These women answered the same set of questions as the group in Chapter 9, the women who wanted VBACs but ended up with repeat cesareans.

Repeat-Cesarean Questions

10. Your age when had repeat cesarean. Same doctor or different one second time around? Same or different hospital?

11. Choose one of the following to best describe your feelings about having a cesarean again. (a) I was certain I wanted to try a VBAC and did. (b) I wanted to try a VBAC but my doctor wouldn't go along with it. (c) I was certain I wanted to have an elective repeat cesarean because . . . please explain. (d) I was ambivalent and had a hard time deciding. Please elaborate on any of these answers if you'd like.

12. How did your doctor influence your decision? Did you at any time negotiate with your doctor? (For example, say you'd try a VBAC if your baby wasn't two weeks late and 9 lbs. like your first one, or you'd try a VBAC if you could have epidural anesthesia?)

13. What actually happened? Did you have an elective repeat cesarean, did you try to have a VBAC, or did something else occur?

14. What was the baby's condition at birth?

15. How long did you stay in the hospital? Any trouble bonding with the baby?

16. How did your recovery compare to the recovery from your first C-section? Any complications?

17. Was the second cesarean easier or harder overall than the first one?

18. If you had it to do over again, which birth option would you choose, cesarean or vaginal birth?

Certainty or Ambivalence?

Ten of the sixteen mothers said they were certain they wanted a repeat cesarean (choice c). Four said they were ambivalent (choice d), and the remaining two said they had wanted to try a VBAC, but then something happened.

Among the ten who were certain about wanting an elective cesarean, five said, in almost identical wording, that they did not want to risk going through labor again only to end up with another cesarean.

"I had such a terrible first birth experience that I wasn't willing to take the chance of the same thing happening again," wrote Jan of Algonquin, Illinois. Her first experience included loss of consciousness after an epidural was administered, a substantial disagreement between attendants as to how far she was dilated when

Pitocin was administered (4 versus 9 centimeters), a great deal of physical pain, postpartum depression, and a feeling that her care was so badly handled that "it was probably grounds for further examination legally." In addition to fearing a repeat of her first experience, there was a possibility she had placenta previa in her second pregnancy, which ruled out vaginal birth.

"I didn't want to go through labor and then be told hours later that a C-section was necessary," echoed Yvonne of Chicago.

Some of the five women added other comments to their answer. "We have a history of large babies, and I did not want to go through labor again just to end up with a C-section in the end," wrote Talia of Glenview, Illinois. She also said, as mentioned in Chapter 7, that she did not "need the experience of a vaginal delivery to make my life whole."

Stephanie of Pacific Palisades, California, also wrote, "I didn't want to be all stretched out vaginally if I chose a VBAC after already having been cut from the C-section."

Meredith of Evanston, Illinois, said that the combination of labor plus surgery is hard on both baby and mother and makes recovery more difficult. In addition, she brought up the controversial "convenience factor" (see Chapter 5, page 87). "I was two weeks late with the first one, and I liked the idea that this would be planned and early," she wrote. "I have a two-year-old, and my family all live out of town so it was nice knowing when the baby was coming."

The convenience issue, at least for the purposes of this book, could be renamed the "help and support" issue. Other women mentioned it in their responses—almost in shame, with comments such as "I hate to admit it"—but what all of them seem to be expressing is a need for help. Suppose a woman was the sole caregiver for her two-year-old. What if nobody was available at the spur of the moment to stay with the toddler when she went to the hospital? What if a woman's husband couldn't take time off to stay home even a few days? What if a woman needed help, without any advance notice, and no relative or friend was there for her? The extended familial support network available to past generations does not exist for many of today's new mothers. In addition, hospital stays of one week or longer in the past allowed mothers to really recuperate before going home. When a new mother is sent home after one or two days, as is customary today, she is barely capable of caring for herself, much less a newborn and another child. Most insurance companies do not cover home-care visits, and, in effect, society ignores the problem.

The other five women who said they were certain they wanted a repeat cesarean offered a variety of reasons.

Doris of Briarcliff Manor, New York, had her first cesarean because she had conceived twins after undergoing in vitro fertilization, and only one fetus was alive at the time the surgery was scheduled. She became pregnant a second time at age forty-one without fertility aids and chose another cesarean, she said, because she "knew what to expect." This feeling, too, was expressed by others, including Stephanie, who said, "I felt comfortable with what I had already experienced with a cesarean, and a vaginal birth was still a foreign experience to me."

Lindsay of Los Angeles, wrote that, for her, having surgery was physically easier than going through labor. She had labored more than twenty hours in her first pregnancy, and dilated to 7 centimeters, but the baby had shown signs of distress, and the doctor didn't want to administer Pitocin for fear the baby wouldn't tolerate it well. In contrast to the labor experience, surgery, she wrote, "was easy—*much* easier than labor with regard to both pain and the long term toll on my body."

One woman gave two reasons for choosing an elective cesarean at age forty-one, not to mention her first cesarean and her second cesarean following a VBAC attempt. When fully dilated and pushing during her VBAC attempt, Julia (Chapter 9) had felt that her previous scar was tearing. And in fact, after the third delivery, her doctor advised her against having any more children because her uterus was "paper thin." Though she suspected this, she did not know it for certain until after the third delivery. But both of her first two babies had weighed more than 9 pounds, and both of her cesareans were done for failure to progress after she had dilated fully and pushed. "I had tried my best to deliver them vaginally and was absolutely certain that it wasn't possible."

The remaining two women who were certain they wanted an elective cesarean both gave cephalopelvic disproportion as the reason. One, Sandra, had been x-rayed during her first labor for the resultant CPD diagnosis. She very much wanted to deliver vaginally in her second pregnancy but did not because the baby was late and bigger than the first. By the third (and fourth) babies, she no longer had a burning desire to experience vaginal delivery.

Likewise, Meg of Fort Worth had not been able to deliver vaginally the first time, she said, because her pelvic opening was too small. She had dilated to 9 centimeters with Pitocin, to no avail. The baby had been born with a congenital condition called a diaphragmatic hernia. He had no left lung and only part of the right lung, and he only lived sixteen hours. Meg did not discuss the emotional effects of losing an infant, which may well have played a part in her subsequent decision to choose a cesarean. She merely wrote, "It wasn't hard to recover [from the surgery], and I knew my pelvis wouldn't widen for a birth." She subsequently gave birth to two healthy babies by repeat cesarean.

Of the four women who said they were ambivalent about which birth option they preferred, one, Shannon of Arlington Heights, Illinois, had given birth by cesarean the first time after twenty-four hours of "extremely painful" labor, augmented by Pitocin, at the end of which she had dilated less than 3 centimeters. All of her babies, she wrote, had very large heads. She felt ambivalent about what to do in the second pregnancy but the second baby, like the first one, was two weeks late. She went into labor at 1:00 A.M, seven hours before her scheduled cesarean.

"At the hospital, the doctor asked if I would like to try a VBAC or have a cesarean," Shannon, a stand-up comedian, wrote. "I said I preferred a third alternative. Oh well. At the onset of labor, I was very insecure because of the first baby, so I decided with little coaxing that I wanted a C-section. So much for the third alternative."

Chris of Oak Park said, "I wanted a VBAC and my doctor was ready and willing—*but* we were equally concerned about a repeat performance." She had been cared for by midwives at a teaching hospital and had given birth by cesarean to a 10 pound 3 ounce boy after three days of unproductive labor, augmented by Pitocin on the third day. She had dilated a total of 1 centimeter in that time. "I was having severe back labor, and we seemed to be getting nowhere fast! Through this whole thing, the baby was fine."

In the second pregnancy, Chris, her husband, and her doctor at a different hospital decided to monitor the baby's weight and let that guide their decision. During the last two months of her pregnancy, Chris wrote, "We *all* equally agreed to a scheduled C-section." Ultrasounds showed the baby weighing in at about 9 pounds. When she delivered him, one week early, he weighed 8 pounds 10 ounces.

Lynette of Norfolk, Virginia, said she had a hard time deciding what to do. Her cesarean for a breech presentation had been done under general anesthesia after five unsuccessful attempts to administer an epidural. By that time she had gone through labor and dilated fully, and the baby had passed meconium and was experiencing worrisome decelerations. "I knew I did not want to repeat the first delivery scene," she wrote, echoing the reasoning of the first five women.

The fourth of the uncertain women, Charlene, said she was ambivalent at first but decided elective cesarean was the best option. She had her first cesarean for failure to progress, and her VBAC attempt with baby number two also ended in cesarean for failure to progress. She, too, had a tendency to produce large babies. She and her doctor discussed various options and she ended up giving birth by cesarean nine days before her due date.

Two women, Casey of Coronado, California, and Kelly of Houston, said they had wanted to try a VBAC. Kelly, whose first baby was breech, said she and her doctor had planned for a VBAC but when baby number two was overdue, she had a cesarean.

Casey changed her mind about wanting a VBAC about one month before her due date. She had experienced a nonprogressive labor with a 9 pound baby girl, in which she had dilated only 1 centimeter after twenty-four hours of labor augmented by Pitocin. "Not until she started showing fetal stress did he [her doctor at a public hospital] recommend a C-section," Casey wrote.

She attributed her change of heart in the second pregnancy to her fear of having another nonprogressive labor, but she also brought up the "help and support" issue. "I knew I would have more than enough help with the baby if I elected to have a C-section." After the surgery, during which she also had a tubal ligation, she said she had an easy recovery because "I took my time about moving around too quickly—I had three adults taking care of the baby for a three-week period!"

How Did Your Caregiver Influence Your Decision?

Most of the sixteen women in the repeat-cesarean group described partnerships with their doctors that involved discussions about various birth scenarios, including the VBAC option. Three women clearly had patient-directed relationships, saying their doctors did what they asked.

None of the women were pressured by their doctors to have surgery simply because they had had it before; only one, Jan, said her doctor pushed for cesarean, because she had placenta previa early in her pregnancy and he was uncertain about the placenta's position later. But this relationship was clearly a partnership; Jan described her doctor as very understanding and eager to find out what had happened in her first pregnancy.

Some of the women described their interactions with their doctors in detail, and they also did some negotiating. Charlene said her doctor presented "two realistic options": to induce two weeks early and try to deliver a baby in the 7-pound range, or to schedule an elective cesarean. "I did not think the first was a very good choice because I was not confident that an induction would be successful, and I thought I would end up with a C-section anyway," she reasoned. "With the first choice, I would have to go through labor, which is tiring, and would have had the baby when it was smaller (and fussier)."

For Chris, the pivotal point in negotiating with her doctor was the baby's size. "My doctor would have attempted a VBAC if I'd requested it," she wrote. "His only concern was repeating what had happened with baby number one—a *very* real concern. I did not want to induce early (at a lower weight) because it had been useless before and I hated the feeling of a 'useless' labor. It had exhausted me, and, I felt, for naught."

Casey's doctor was not quite as flexible. "He agreed to perform the section," she wrote, "but with the condition that we wait two weeks after my due date, in case I would be able to go into labor for a VBAC." Casey didn't go into labor, and her son was delivered by cesarean. He weighed 11 pounds 7 ounces.

Several women praised their doctors, more so than did women in the other groups. "My doctor was very good in not swaying my decision either way," wrote Talia. "She also let me know, I shouldn't feel guilty about not even trying a normal delivery first."

Meredith liked both her doctors and delivered both her babies at her town's university teaching hospital. But she appreciated one major difference between the two doctors. At the six-week checkup following her first cesarean, which was done for failure to progress after attempts with Pitocin caused heart-rate decelerations, her first doctor explained that what had happened would not necessarily recur and that Meredith would be a good candidate for VBAC. There was nothing wrong with this information, but Meredith sensed immediately that he "was going to spend all nine months of my next pregnancy talking me into having a vaginal birth." Yet she already felt she would want an elective cesarean, because, like so many other women, she was "afraid to go through hours of labor only to have a C-section anyway."

The second doctor, a woman practicing at the same hospital, made sure Meredith knew about the VBAC option, then left it at that. "Her response to my wanting another C-section was that the important thing is that the decision is mine," Meredith wrote. "Not a lot of physicians feel that way." The new doctor asked her at each monthly visit whether she still wanted a cesarean, and Meredith's response was always the same. "The only time that I negotiated with her was when I told her that if I went into labor before the due date that *maybe* I would try a VBAC," she wrote. "I only mentioned it once. I was 99.9 percent sure that I wanted to have a C-section."

An observed difference between this group and the women who preferred VBACs but had a cesarean is that half of the women in this group stayed with the same doctor, whereas most of the women who attempted a VBAC had a different doctor. Though no numerical conclusions can be drawn from this, it is possible that the same doctor could make a better clinical assessment of an individual woman's chances at VBAC than a doctor who bases his or her medical recommendation on the patient's written records, which never tell the entire story. The same doctor could also better appreciate a woman's emotional responses to her first cesarean (if the doctor cares to) and perhaps better empathize with the reasons for her choice.

What Happened?

All sixteen women had repeat cesareans; in answering question 13, most simply wrote that they had a scheduled cesarean. A couple of women who had weighed the option of inducing early to try to have a smaller baby commented that they were glad they hadn't pursued that.

Charlene had considered her doctor's suggestion of inducing two weeks early in the hope of delivering a 7-pound baby. Instead, she had the cesarean nine days before the due date and still gave birth to an 8 pound 12 ounce baby. "Even if I had tried an induction two weeks early," she wrote, "the baby probably would have been too big."

Likewise, Chris had her cesarean one week before the due date, when an ultrasound estimated his weight (accurately!) at 9 pounds. Her first son had weighed 10 pounds 3 ounces

"He ended up weighing 8 lbs. 10 oz. at birth," she wrote. "But this time, I was fully aware and there for everything. It was wonderful."

How Was the Baby at Birth?

All the women in the elective-cesarean group gave birth to healthy babies. There were two meconium deliveries, and one of the babies, Talia's, had to be intubated to have the meconium removed. As we have seen, this can happen in vaginal or cesarean deliveries. "Luckily it was not too serious and didn't take long to take care of," she wrote. "Other than that she was fine."

The other meconium delivery was that of Casey, who gave birth to an 11 pound 7 ounce boy two weeks past her due date (at her doctor's insistence). "He was big and healthy, although it was a meconium delivery, so there was a little concern at birth," she wrote.

The baby belonging to Meredith was born with a little fluid in his lungs, which is more common in cesarean deliveries than vaginal deliveries. However, the baby was not premature and did not have respiratory distress; he simply had to be observed. "It did not happen with the first, so I was surprised but not alarmed," Meredith wrote. "They let my husband hold him for only a short period of time and then they took him right to the nursery. He was then in my room four hours later and doing fine."

All the other women answered "perfect," "excellent," "great," or something synonymous to this question. None of the women said they had trouble bonding with their baby.

How Was Your Recovery?

Hospital stays have gotten shorter, and not just for vaginal deliveries. The shortest stay in the elective-cesarean group was thirty-six hours. The mother, Lynette, an emergency-room nurse, said "I felt great, I felt so good, I just wanted to get home. I had no nurse or family other than my husband, who took off a day or two. I felt so good I could have gone back to work in three weeks."

Lynette was pleasantly surprised by her second recovery because she had prepared herself psychologically for a much harder time. In the first delivery, she had come to the hospital 10 centimeters dilated, with a baby in breech position, "ready to go." But there were two simultaneous trauma events in the hospital's emergency room, and Lynette had to wait ninety minutes for anesthesia. When the anesthesiologists finally got to her, they made five unsuccessful attempts to give her an epidural. The baby began to have decelerations, and Lynette had to go under general anesthesia. She described the experience as "hideous."

The circumstances were much different and more under control for her elective repeat and, when everything went well, she was euphoric. In addition, she said, "I had very little post-op pain because I had long-acting epidural morphine," which she hadn't had the first time. Her first thirty-six hours were nearly pain free.

Chris stayed five days in the hospital but also commented that keeping the epidural in place for several days made a huge difference in her recovery. "I never took a painkiller (orally), not Tylenol—nothing!" she wrote. "I think that that, singly, eased the pain, which eased the recovery. I was up quickly and was in bed at home for only a few days (due to my mom mostly)."

Despite the greater availability of high-tech pain relief, which may enhance recovery, the other women stayed a range of between two and six days in the hospital. Still, there's definitely a movement to discharge women more quickly. And there's somewhat of an irony attached to this debate. On average, women who have an elective cesarean without complications may stay three days; those who have a successful VBAC without complications may stay only two days. But those who go through labor and then end up with another cesarean must stay the longest, usually four to six days. So there is some financial risk-taking involved in promoting VBAC—health care dollars are saved by the 60 to 80 percent who succeed but are lost by the other 20 to 40 percent who end up with a repeat cesarean.

As an example of the latter, Julia of Los Angeles, stayed in the hospital only three days after her elective cesarean, but she stayed six and five days for the two preceding operations, both of which had occurred after full labor.

Still, if saving dollars is the main goal, persuading everybody who is eligible to attempt VBAC makes financial sense because the odds favor success. Unfortunately, saving money is the only incentive behind forcing women to leave the hospital early. And it is not a sound policy.

Sandra, for instance, stayed five nights after her first cesarean in 1987 but only two nights after her fourth cesarean (elective) in 1995 at the same hospital. For her, the two-day stay was too short. "It was one day less than I needed," she wrote. "The first night home was only sixty hours after the surgery and my body still had a lot of pain when I moved. I still needed a nurse to bring baby number 4 to me in bed, a task that I couldn't ask my husband to constantly do while he cared for our other three children. After a week, however, the recovery was a breeze."

Nine women reported having easier recoveries with this cesarean (question 16), six said recovery was similar, and one said it was more difficult. Likewise, in answering question 17, nine women said the second cesarean was easier overall, five said there was no difference, and two said it was harder.

In responding to the second part of question 16 (any complications?), four women cited minor problems, all relating to drugs, either anesthesia or painkillers. No women reported fever, infection, or the need for a transfusion.

Several of the women who reported easier recoveries, including Charlene and Julia, said they were better rested after surgery because they hadn't gone through an exhausting labor.

Jan, who had had a "terrible" experience the first time, called this birth a "pleasant" event by comparison.

The one woman who said recovery was harder, Meredith, attributed it to the demands of her two-year-old. "It was difficult to keep her off my lap and I could not rest much," she wrote. "I had one bad day after getting out of the hospital and by two weeks I was back to normal."

Meredith was also one of two women who said the second cesarean (not just the recovery) was harder overall. While most people said they were reassured by knowing what to expect, this aspect had the reverse effect on Meredith. In her first delivery, she wrote, everything had happened so fast that she didn't have time to react or think about it. The second time she walked calmly into a hospital room, got an IV and catheter, and walked into the operating room. "The spinal hurt this time, and I was terrified after I laid down and they started cleaning my stomach," she wrote. "The cutting took a long time, because they had to cut through my previous scar. I could feel pressure when they pulled him out, and that was strange. Basically, I was much more aware of what was going on, and I did not love it." Afterward, however, she felt better, "because the first time I had been up the night before and then in labor all day so I was completely exhausted."

The other woman who said the second cesarean was harder complained that she could feel too much. "I felt it when she went in to cut me, and when she took my baby out I thought she pulled the life out of me," Yvonne of Chicago wrote. By contrast, when she had her third cesarean, the doctors and nurses were "wonderful," and she didn't feel any pain.

In addition to Yvonne's contention that her epidural was not strong enough, there were three other drug-related complaints. The most serious came from Casey, who said that a headache from her spinal anesthesia added a fifth day to her hospital stay. "The second section was performed with a spinal (although I strongly requested an epidural,)" she wrote. "The needle hole took longer to close, which allowed air to enter, causing headaches." Nonetheless, Casey still described the second cesarean as "easy—physically and mentally."

Sandra complained of itching from the morphine she had received for pain after all four of her operations. And Stephanie said she had a sensitivity to both the epidural and the Demoral she received. "Drugs and I don't mix well," she explained.

As a whole, however, the women in this group fared well and had no serious difficulties with their recoveries.

What Would You Do If You Had Another Baby?

Question 18 asked women which birth option they would choose if they had another baby. Fourteen of the sixteen women wrote "cesarean."

Of the remaining two, Lynette just wrote, "I wish I had the nerve to try vaginal." It wasn't labor that she feared, having gone through it once, but the possibility of another "uncontrolled situation."

Yvonne said she would prefer a vaginal delivery because "recovery is easier," but she would ultimately choose whichever method proves best for the baby because "baby comes first."

· · · · · ·

Conclusions

If any salient conclusions can be drawn from the experiences of the fifty women surveyed here, they might include those below.

Women for whom fast recovery from childbirth was paramount tended to choose VBAC. These women did not seem to fear labor, even a very long labor. Similarly, as a group, they seemed less preoccupied with the potential ill effects of prolonged labor on the baby than the women who chose elective cesarean. They embraced the idea that vaginal birth is normal, that nature intended it to be that way. Many, but not all, wanted to labor without pain relief.

Many of the women who chose VBAC viewed themselves as capable of meeting the challenge of pushing the baby out of their body and into the world. Some of them exclaimed, "I did it!"—an indication that they viewed vaginal birth as a victory, or an accomplishment above and beyond their first cesarean delivery.

Conversely, women who chose elective cesarean wanted to take the uncertainties of labor out of the equation. What they universally feared the most was a repetition of the first experience, in which they had typically labored for a long time, without adequate progress, sometimes without adequate pain relief, only to end up with a cesarean. (Even though some of the women who chose VBAC had a similar first experience, it did not seem to bother them as much.) The elective cesarean women were eager to take advantage of the available measures to eliminate pain and still be awake for the delivery, courtesy of epidural or spinal anesthesia. (None wanted a general anesthesia.) They were more willing to endure the pain of recovery from surgery than the pain of labor, possibly because recovery is theirs alone and cannot harm the baby.

In addition, the length of the recovery period was not an issue for them. They were willing to pull out all the medical stops to achieve what they perceived as a safe delivery for their baby, even if it meant a longer recovery. As one woman put it, they did not need the experience of vaginal birth to make them feel whole. Most felt that giving birth to a healthy infant was a significant accomplishment, regardless of the method.

Overall, the women who seemed happiest were the ones who *knew* what they wanted and *got* what they wanted. Kathy was very happy with her two VBACs, despite the fact that she broke her coccyx pushing out the last baby. Sandra was happy with her elective repeat cesareans once she had talked herself out of the feeling of failure after the primary cesarean.

Even some of the women who wanted to have a VBAC, but for some reason could not—such as Sonia, who pushed for three hours and still ended up with a cesarean—said they would try VBAC again. I believe this is because it is clearly their choice to try a VBAC, and they know they could cope with the consequences if it did not work.

However, the women who were ambivalent about VBAC in the first place (and were perhaps persuaded by their doctors) were less delighted with the outcome, especially if it was a repeat cesarean, but even to some degree if the VBAC worked.

What I conclude from these stories is that it is best to have a plan that is yours, not somebody else's. Along those lines, I would like to leave you with something written by Chris, one of the mothers in the survey.

"To me the birth process is analogous to a wedding. There are different options in *how* you get married, but the significant part is the marriage. In the birth process, there are also options, but the most important part is having a healthy baby and raising it! The birth is just the beginning!"

Bibliography

Chapter 1. *The Drive to Lower the Cesarean Rate*

American College of Obstetricians and Gynecologists, *ACOG Committee Opinion*, 143, October 1994, "Vaginal Delivery After a Previous Cesarean Birth."

American College of Obstetricians and Gynecologists, *ACOG Practice Patterns*, 1, August 1995, "Vaginal Delivery After Previous Cesarean Birth." (Clinical practice guidelines for issues in obstetrics and gynecology.)

American College of Obstetricians and Gynecologists, Statement on Cesarean Delivery, May 18, 1994.

Centers for Disease Control and Prevention, *Morbidity and Mortality Weekly Report (MMWR)*, 44, no. 15, April 21, 1995.

Columbia University College of Physicians and Surgeons Complete Guide to Pregnancy, Donald F. Tapley, M.D., et al., eds. Crown Publishers, New York, 1988.

Cunningham, F. Gary, M.D., et al. *Williams Obstetrics,* 19th Edition, Appleton and Lange, Norwalk, Connecticut, 1993.

Flamm, Bruce, M.D. "Cesarean Delivery 1970-1995: Where Have We Been and Where Are We Going?" *International Journal of Childbirth Education,* November 1994.

Gabay, Mary, and Sidney M. Wolfe, M.D. *Unnecessary Cesarean Sections: Curing a National Epidemic*, Public Citizen's Health Research Group, 1994. (This book can be ordered from Public Citizen's Health Research Group, Publications Dept., 1600 20th St. NW, Washington, D.C. 20009-1001. Phone: 202-588-1000.)

National Center for Health Statistics, *Monthly Vital Statistics Report,* 43, no. 5 (S), October 25, 1994.

Parrish, Kiyoko M., Ph.D., et al. "Effect of Changes in Maternal Age, Parity, and Birth Weight Distribution on Primary Cesarean Delivery Rates." *Journal of the American Medical Association,* 271, no. 6, February 9, 1994.

Petitti, Diana B., M.D. "The Epidemiology of Fetal Death." *Clinical Obstetrics and Gynecology,* 30, no. 2, June 1987.

Porreco, Richard, M.D. Telephone interview with the director of perinatal services, Columbia-Health One (a group of hospitals) in Denver, Colorado, and associate clinical professor of ob-gyn at University of Colorado Health Sciences Center. July 1995.

Socol, Michael L, M.D. Personal interview with professor and head, section of maternal-fetal medicine, department of obstetrics and gynecology, Northwestern University Medical School, Chicago, Illinois. March 1993.

Tulsky, Alex, M.D. Telephone interview with retired ob-gyn in Chicago, medical historian. October 1995.

Chapter 2. The Medical Reasons for Cesarean Delivery

American College of Obstetricians and Gynecologists. *ACOG Committee Opinion,* 143, October 1994, "Vaginal Delivery After a Previous Cesarean Birth."

American College of Obstetricians and Gynecologists. *ACOG Practice Patterns,* 1, August 1995, "Vaginal Delivery After Previous Cesarean Birth." (Clinical practice guidelines for issues in obstetrics and gynecology.)

American College of Obstetricians and Gynecologists, Statement on Cesarean Delivery, May 18, 1994.

Centers for Disease Control and Prevention, *Morbidity and Mortality Weekly Report (MMWR),* 44, no. 4, February 3, 1995.

Cunningham, F. Gary, M.D., et al. *Williams Obstetrics,* 19th Edition, Appleton and Lange, Norwalk, Connecticut, 1993.

Gabay, Mary and Sidney M. Wolfe, M.D. *Unnecessary Cesarean Sections: Curing a National Epidemic,* Public Citizen's Health Research Group, 1994.

López-Zeno, José A., M.D., et al. "A Controlled Trial of a Program for the Active Management of Labor." *New England Journal of Medicine,* 326, no. 7, February 13, 1992.

Marx, Phyllis D., M.D. Written correspondence.

National Center for Health Statistics, *Monthly Vital Statistics Report,* 44, no. 3 (S), September 21, 1995.

Phelan, Jeffrey P., M.D., moderator of symposium; Steven L. Clark, M.D., Richard P. Porreco, M.D., and J. Peter Van Dorsten, M.D., panelists; "Finding Alternatives to Cesarean Section." *Contemporary Ob/Gyn,* January 1988.

Chapter 3. The Facts About VBAC

American College of Obstetricians and Gynecologists. *ACOG Committee Opinion,* 143, October 1994, "Vaginal Delivery After a Previous Cesarean Birth."

American College of Obstetricians and Gynecologists. *ACOG Practice Patterns*, 1, August 1995, "Vaginal Delivery After Previous Cesarean Birth." (Clinical practice guidelines for issues in obstetrics and gynecology.)

Baquet, Dean and Jane Fritsch. "New York's Public Hospitals Fail, and Babies are the Victims." *The New York Times*, March 5, 1995.

Baquet, Dean and Jane Fritsch. "Lack of Oversight Takes Delivery-Room Toll." *The New York Times*, March 6, 1995.

Baquet, Dean and Jane Fritsch. "In Chaotic City Hospitals, a Bureaucracy to Match." *The New York Times*, March 7, 1995.

Bowes, Watson, M.D. Telephone interview with professor, department of obstetrics and gynecology, University of North Carolina, Chapel Hill, November 1995.

Centers for Disease Control and Prevention, *Morbidity and Mortality Weekly Report (MMWR)*, 44, no. 15, April 21, 1995.

Chazotte, Cynthia, M.D., Robert Madden, Ph.D., and Wayne R. Cohen, M.D., "Labor Patterns in Women with Previous Cesareans." *Obstetrics and Gynecology*, 75, no. 3, Part 1, March 1990.

Cunningham, F. Gary, M.D., et al. *Williams Obstetrics*, 19th Edition, Appleton and Lange, Norwalk, Connecticut, 1993.

Eisenberg, Arlene, Heidi E. Murkoff, and Sandee E. Hathaway, *What to Expect When You're Expecting*, 2nd edition, Workman Publishing, New York, 1991.

Flamm, Bruce L., M.D., and Janice R. Goings, R.N., CNM. "Vaginal Birth After Cesarean Section: Is Suspected Fetal Macrosomia a Contraindication?" *Obstetrics and Gynecology*, 74, no. 5, November 1989.

Flamm, Bruce L., M.D., et al. "Vaginal Birth After Cesarean Delivery: Results of a 5-Year Multicenter Collaborative Study." *Obstetrics and Gynecology*, 76, no. 5, Part 1, November 1990.

Gabay, Mary and Sidney M. Wolfe, M.D. *Unnecessary Cesarean Sections: Curing a National Epidemic,* Public Citizens's Health Research Group, 1994.

Goldman, Gail, BSc, et al. "Factors Influencing the Practice of Vaginal Birth after Cesarean Section." *American Journal of Public Health*, 83, no. 8, August 1993.

Hale, Ralph, M.D. "Reducing the Rate of Cesarean Deliveries/An Obtainable but Elusive Goal." *Journal of the American Medical Association*, 272, no. 7, August 17, 1994.

Harlass, Frederick E., M.D., and Patrick Duff, M.D. "The Duration of Labor in Primiparas Undergoing Vaginal Birth After Cesarean Delivery." *Obstetrics and Gynecology*, 75, no. 1, January 1990.

King, Dale E., M.A., and Kajal Lahiri, Ph.D. "Socioeconomic Factors and the Odds of Vaginal Birth After Cesarean Delivery." *Journal of the Ameican Medical Association,* 272, No. 7, August 17, 1994.

Morgan, Mark A., M.D., and Gary R. Thurnau, M.D. "Efficacy of the Fetal-Pelvic Index for Delivery of Neonates Weighing 4000 Grams or Greater: A Preliminary Report." *American Journal of Obstetrics and Gynecology,* 158, no. 5, May 1988.

National Center for Health Statistics. *Monthly Vital Statistics Report,* 44, no. 3 (S), September 21, 1995.

Ollendorff, David A., M.D., et al. "Vaginal Birth after Cesarean Section for Arrest of Labor: Is Success Determined by Maximum Cervical Dilatation during the Prior Labor?" *American Journal of Obstetrics and Gynecology,* 159, no. 3, September 1988.

Rosen, Mortimer G., M.D., and Janet C. Dickinson, BSN, MSW. "Vaginal Birth after Cesarean: A Meta-analysis of Indicators for Success." *Obstetrics and Gynecology,* 76, no. 5, Part 1, November 1990.

Stafford, Randall S., Ph.D. "The Impact of Nonclinical Factors on Repeat Cesarean Section." *Journal of the American Medical Association,* 265, no. 1, January 2, 1991.

Thurnau, Gary R., M.D., Kurt A. Hales, M.D., and Mark A. Morgan, M.D. "Evaluation of the Fetal-Pelvic Relationship." *Clinical Obstetrics and Gynecology,* 35, no. 3, September 1992.

Thurnau, Gary R., M.D., David H. Scates, M.D., and Mark A. Morgan, M.D. "The Fetal-Pelvic Index: A Method of Identifying Fetal-Pelvic Disproportion in Women Attempting Vaginal Birth after Previous Cesarean delivery." *American Journal of Obstetrics and Gynecology,* 165, no. 2, August 1991.

Thurnau, Gary R., M.D. Telephone interview with professor, department of obstetrics and gynecology, section of maternal fetal medicine, and director of the Prenatal Assessment Center at the University of Oklahoma Health Sciences Center College of Medicine in Oklahoma City, Oklahoma. May 1995.

Troyer, Lisa R., M.D., and Valerie M. Parisi,, M.D., MPH. "Obstetric Parameters Affecting Success in a Trial of Labor: Designation of a Scoring System," *American Journal of Obstetrics and Gynecology,* 167, no. 4, Part 1, October 1992.

Chapter 4. Weighing the Risks

Abitbol, M. Maurice, et al. "Maternal Complications Following Prolonged or

Arrested Labor." Journal of Maternal-Fetal Investigation, 4:9-13, 1994.

American College of Obstetricians and Gynecologists. ACOG Committee Opinion, 143, October 1994, "Vaginal Delivery After a Previous Cesarean Birth."

American College of Obstetricians and Gynecologists. ACOG Practice Patterns 1, August 1995, "Vaginal Delivery After Previous Cesarean Birth." (Clinical practice guidelines for issues in obstetrics and gynecology.)

Atrash, Hani, M.D. Telephone interview with chief of the pregnancy and infant health branch at the Centers for Disease Control and Prevention. November 1995.

Cowan, Robert K., M.D., et al. "Trial of Labor Following Cesarean Delivery," Obstetrics and Gynecology, 83, no. 6, June 1994.

Cunningham, F. Gary, M.D., et al. Williams Obstetrics, 19th Edition, Appleton and Lange, Norwalk, Connecticut, 1993.

Farmer, Richard M., M.D., Ph.D., et al. "Uterine Rupture during Trial of Labor after Previous Cesarean Section." American Journal of Obstetrics and Gynecology, 165, no. 4, Part I, October 1991.

Flamm, Bruce L., M.D., and Janice R. Goings, R.N., CNM. "Vaginal Birth After Cesarean Section: Is Suspected Fetal Macrosomia a Contraindication?" Obstetrics and Gynecology, 74, no. 5, November 1989.

Flamm, Bruce L., M.D., et al. "Elective Repeat Cesarean Delivery Versus Trial of Labor: A Prospective Multicenter Study." Obstetrics and Gynecology, 83, no. 6, June 1994.

Flamm, Bruce L., M.D., et al. "Vaginal Birth After Cesarean Delivery: Results of a 5-Year Multicenter Collaborative Study." Obstetrics and Gynecology, 76, no. 5, Part 1, November 1990.

Flamm, Bruce, M.D. Telephone interview with research chairman for the Kaiser Permanente Medical Group in Southern California and assistant clinical professor of obstetrics and gynecology at the University of California. July 1995.

Hadley, Carolyn, M.D., Michael T. Mennuti, M.D., and Steven G. Gabbe, M.D. "An Evaluation of the Relative Risks of a Trial of Labor Versus Elective Repeat Cesarean Section," American Journal of Perinatology, 3, no. 2, April 1986.

Iffy, Leslie, M.D. Telephone interview with professor, department of obstetrics and gynecology at the New Jersey Medical School in Newark, New Jersey. July 1995.

Jones, Richard O., M.D., et al. "Rupture of Low Transverse Cesarean Scars During Trial of Labor." Obstetrics and Gynecology, 77, no. 6, June 1991.

Leung, Anna S., M.D., et al. "Risk Factors Associated with Uterine Rupture during Trial of Labor after Cesarean Delivery: A Case-control Study." *American Journal of Obstetrics and Gynecology,* 168, no. 5, May 1993.

McCann, Sheila. "FHP Must Pay Disabled Boy $8 Million/Jury Award for Tot Born Brain-Damaged Sets a Record for Utah's State Court." *Salt Lake Tribune,* January 28, 1993.

Meehan, Fergus P., MAO, FRCOG, MSc, et al. "Delivery Following Cesarean Section and Perinatal Mortality." *American Journal of Perinatology,* 6, No. 1, January 1989.

Meier, Paul R., M.D., and Richard P. Porreco, M.D. "Trial of Labor Following Cesarean Section: A Two-year Experience," *American Journal of Obstetrics and Gynecology,* 144, no. 6, November 15, 1982.

National Center for Health Statistics. *Monthly Vital Statistics Report,* 43, no. 6 (S), March 22, 1995.

Rosen, Mortimer, M.D., Janet C. Dickinson, BSN, MSW, and Carolyn L. Westhoff, M.D., MSc. "Vaginal Birth after Cesarean: A Meta-analysis of Morbidity and Mortality." *Obstetrics and Gynecology,* 77, no. 3, March 1991.

Schoendorf, Ken, M.D., MPH. Telephone interview with medical epidemiologist, infant and child health studies branch, National Center for Health Statistics, Centers for Disease Control and Prevention. November 1995.

Scott, James, M.D. Telephone interview with chairman, department of obstetrics and gynecology, University of Utah Medical Center, Salt Lake City, Utah, phone interview, July 1995.

Scott, James, M.D. "Mandatory Trial of Labor After Cesarean Delivery: An Alternative Viewpoint." *Obstetrics and Gynecology,* 77, no. 6, June 1991.

Stone, Joanne, M.D., et al. "Morbidity of failed labor in patients with prior cesarean section." *American Journal of Obstetrics and Gynecology,* 167, no. 6, December 1992.

Yetman, Thomas, M.D., and Thomas E. Nolan, M.D., "Vaginal Birth after Cesarean Section: A Reappraisal of Risk," *American Journal of Obstetrics & Gynecology,* 161, no. 5, November 1989.

Chapter 5. Why Half of Mothers Prefer Surgery

Abitbol, M. Maurice, M.D. Telephone interview with chairman, department of obstetrics and gynecology, Jamaica Hospital Medical Center, Jamaica, New York, and clinical associate professor of obstetrics and gynecology, State University of New York. April 1995.

Abitbol, M. Maurice, M.D., (Editorial) "A Further View on the VBAC Quandary." *American Family Physician,* 47, January 1993.

Abitbol, M. Maurice, M.D., et al. "Vaginal Birth After Cesarean Section: The Patient's Point of View." *American Family Physician,* 47, January 1993.

American College of Obstetricians and Gynecologists. *ACOG Committee Opinion,* 108, May 1992, "Ethical Dimensions of Informed Consent."

American College of Obstetricians and Gynecologists. *ACOG Committee Opinion,* 143, October 1994, "Vaginal Delivery After a Previous Cesarean Birth."

American College of Obstetricians and Gynecologists. *ACOG Practice Patterns* 1, August 1995, "Vaginal Delivery After Previous Cesarean Birth." (Clinical practice guidelines for issues in obstetrics and gynecology.)

Blank, Roneen, M.D. Telephone interview with psychiatrist and clinical director of the perinatal support services program at Good Samaritan Hospital in Downers Grove, Illinois. July 1995.

Butler, Jane, CNM, MPH, et al. "Supportive nurse-midwife care is associated with a reduced incidence of cesarean section." *American Journal of Obstetrics and Gynecology,* 168, no. 5, May 1993.

Cain, Joanna, M.D. Telephone interview with gynecological oncologist, University of Washington at Seattle, and chairman of the ACOG ethics committee. July 1995.

Feldman, George B., M.D., and Freiman, Jennie A., M.D. "Prophylactic Cesarean Section at Term?" *New England Journal of Medicine,* 312, no. 19, May 9, 1985.

Joseph, Gerald F., Jr., M.D., Charles M. Stedman, M.D., and Alfred G. Robichaux, M.D. "Vaginal Birth after Cesarean Section: The Impact of Patient Resistance to a Trial of Labor." *American Journal of Obstetrics and Gynecology,* 164, no. 6, Part 1, June 1991.

Jukelevics, Nicette, M.A. Telephone interview with parent education coordinator in Torrance, California. February 1995.

Kennell, John, M.D., et al. "Continuous Emotional Support During Labor in a U.S. Hospital," *Journal of the American Medical Association,* 265, no. 17, May 1, 1991.

Kirk, E. Paul, M.D., et al. "Vaginal Birth after Cesarean or Repeat Cesarean Section: Medical Risks or Social Realities?" *American Journal of Obstetrics and Gynecology,* 162, no. 6, June 1990.

McClain, Carol Shepherd, Ph.D. "Patient Decision Making: The Case of Delivery Method After a Previous Cesarean Section," *Culture, Medicine, and Psychiatry,* 11, 1987.

McClain, Carol Shepherd, Ph.D. "The Making of a Medical Tradition: Vaginal Birth After Cesarean." *Social Science and Medicine,* 31, no. 2, 1990.

Meier, Paul R., M.D., and Richard P. Porreco, M.D. "Trial of Labor Following Cesarean Section: A Two-year Experience." *American Journal of Obstetrics and Gynecology,* 144, no. 6, November 15, 1982.

Myers, Stephen A., M.D., and Norbert Gleicher, M.D. "A Successful Program to Lower the Cesarean-Section Rates." *New England Journal of Medicine,* 319, no. 23, December 8, 1988.

Chapter 6. Finding the Right Medical Partner

American College of Nurse-Midwives. "Nurse-Midwifery Care of Women Planning a Vaginal Birth After Cesarean (VBAC)." *Clinical Practice Statement,* 1992.

Gabay, Mary, and Sidney M. Wolfe, M.D. *Unnecessary Cesarean Sections: Curing a National Epidemic,* Public Citizen's Health Research Group, 1994.

Korte, Diana and Roberta Scaer. *A Good Birth, A Safe Birth*, 3rd edition, The Harvard Common Press, Harvard and Boston, 1992.

Korte, Diana. *Every Woman's Body*, Ballantine Books, New York, 1994.

Korte, Diana. Telephone interview. February 1995.

Marx, Phyllis D., M.D. Telephone interview. January 1995.

Smith, John M., M.D. Telephone interview. February 1995.

Smith, John M., M.D. *Women and Doctors*, Dell Publishing, New York, 1992.

Chapters 7 through 10

Abitbol, M. Maurice, M.D. Telephone interview with chairman, department of obstetrics and gynecology, Jamaica Hospital Medical Center, Jamaica, New York, and clinical associate professor of obstetrics and gynecology, State University of New York. April 1995.

American College of Nurse-Midwives. Telephone interview. February 1996.

Thurnau, Gary R., M.D. Telephone interview with professor, department of obstetrics and gynecology, section of maternal fetal medicine, and director of the Prenatal Assessment Center at the University of Oklahoma Health Sciences Center College of Medicine in Oklahoma City, Oklahoma. May 1995.

APPENDIX

. . . .

Labor and Delivery Summary

Labor and delivery summaries are designed by hospitals for record keeping purposes. There may be variations in the format, but the information covered is standard. Below are brief explanations of these sections and abbreviations.

When considering whether to attempt VBAC and reflecting on the circumstances of your previous cesarean, you may find it helpful to review your labor and delivery summary. You can request this from the medical records department of the hospital where you delivered.

1. Mother's Delivery History In terms of number of infants. *G* = gravida. *T* = term. *P* = preterm. *A* = abortions. *L* = current live infants.

2. Gestational Information *LMP* = last menstrual period. *LMP EDC* = estimated date of confinement according to LMP. *US EDC* = ultrasound estimated date of confinement. *Assigned GA* = assigned gestational age, in weeks.

3. Complications and Procedures *Other* = this includes any significant medical history which may affect labor and delivery.

4. Labor and Delivery Medications *CLE* = continuous lumbar epidural. Delivery Room Medications often include Pitocin to contract the uterus postpartum.

5. Labor Summary *AROM* = artificial rupture of membranes. *SROM* = spontaneous rupture of membranes. *Complete Dil* = complete dilation.

6. Fetal Data *PG* = prostaglandin, used to ripen cervix. *Laminaria/Dilapan* = used to ripen cervix prior to inducing labor. *AMOL* = active management of labor. *None, IUFD* = none, due to intrauterine fetal demise. *Ext Toco* = external tocodynamometer, a device measuring the force of contractions. *IUPC* = Intrauterine pressure catheter, a more accurate measure of force of contractions.

7. Vaginal Delivery Data *Prior C/S VTOL* = prior cesarean pa-

Labor and Delivery Summary

(1) | G | P | T | A | L | Type and RH |

Private □ Clinic □ Transport □
From: _____

(2) LMP ___/___/___
LMP EDC ___/___/___
US EDC ___/___/___
Assigned GA: ___ wks

COMPLICATIONS/PROCEDURES

(3)
□ Antepartum admission
□ Prenatal care elsewhere
□ No/poor prenatal care

□ Febrile (±100.4°)
□ Suspect amnionitis

□ Abruption
□ Previa, active bleeding
□ Hemorrhage, other
□ Accreta/percreta
□ DIC
□ Platelets d,000

□ Maternal seizure/eclampsia
□ Maternal seizure/other
□ Major anesthetic complication

□ Operative injury, GI
□ Operative injury, GU
□ Uterine inversion
□ Uterine rupture/dehiscence

□ Swan-Ganz
□ Arterial line
□ Amnioinfusion
□ Amniocentesis non-genetic

□ Version prior to labor
□ Scalp pH done
□ Shoulder dystocia
□ Other _____

□ **No complications**

LABOR ANESTHESIA □ None

(4)
□ CLE □ Analgesics
Last Narcotic Prior to Delivery
(med): _____
(dose) (route) (time)

DELIVERY ANESTHESIA

□ None   □ Local/Pudendal
□ CLE   □ Spinal
□ General   □ Other _____

DELIVERY ROOM MEDICATIONS

(med) _____
(dose) (route) (time) (sig)
_____
_____
_____

LABOR SUMMARY **(5)**

Hosp Admit ___/___/___ ___:___
□ AROM
□ SROM   ___/___/___ ___:___
Labor begun ___/___/___ ___:___
Complete Dil ___/___/___ ___:___
Delivery ___/___/___ ___:___
Placenta ___/___/___ ___:___

PRESENTATION **(6)**

□ Vertex   □ Breech, frank
□ Face/brow □ Breech, complete
□ Transverse □ Breech, footling
□ Compound □ Unknown

INDUCTION   □ No □ Yes
□ Oxytocin □ PG □ Other

Initiated ___/___/___ ___:___
□ AROM □ Laminaria/Dilapan

AUGMENTATION □ No □ Yes
□ AMOL
Initiated ___/___/___ ___:___

TERMINATION □ Therapeutic
□ Anomalies □ Other

FHR MONITORING
□ Electronic   □ Auscultation
□ None   □ None, IUFD
□ Ext FHR   □ Int FHR
□ Ext Toco   □ IUPC

DELIVERY DATA—VAGINAL **(7)**

Delivered Prior to Admission □

Prior C/S VTOL □ No □ Yes

VAGINAL CEPHALIC
□ Spontaneous □ Mid forceps
□ Outlet forceps □ MF rotation
□ Low forceps □ Vacuum

VAGINAL BREECH
□ Spontaneous □ Assisted
□ Extraction   □ Forceps AC head

□ EPISIOTOMY   □ None
□ Midline   □ Mediolateral

LACERATIONS   □ None
□ 1° □ 2° □ 3° □ 4°
□ Vaginal   □ Cervical
□ Periurethral

CATHED IN DR
□ No   □ Yes

Most recent HCT: ___ **(8)**

ANTIBIOTICS PRE CORD CLAMP

(9)
□ No □ Yes, Prophylactic
        □ Yes, Therapeutic

DELIVERY DATA—CESAREAN **(10)**

Planned VTOL □ No □ Yes
C/S   □ 1st □ 2nd □ ≥3rd
In labor □ No □ Yes
max dilatation ___ cm

INDICATIONS
1st 2nd
□ □ Planned
□ □ CPD/FTP
□ □ Prior C/S, failed TOL
□ □ Dehiscence/rupture
□ □ Breech
□ □ Other malpres.
□ □ Previa
□ □ Abruptio
□ □ Nonreassuring FHR
         (no/normal scalp pH)
□ □ Nonreassuring FHR
         (low scalp pH)
□ □ Cord prolapse
□ □ Failed trial forceps/
         vacuum
□ □ Other _____

CESAREAN INCISION
□ Low transverse □ Low vertical
□ Classical   □ T-incision
□ Cesarean hysterectomy,
   elective

Foley output: _____

PLACENTA **(11)**
□ Spontaneous □ Expressed
□ Manual   □ Uterus explored
Abnormalities: _____
Path req # : _____

UMBILICAL CORD: 2 3 vessels
□ Nuchal cord □ Cord knot
EBL: _____

TRANSFUSION IN DR □ No
□ Yes, RBC □ Yes, Other

SURGICAL
□ Tubal ligation □ Curettage
□ Hysterectomy, non-elective
□ Other _____

Path req # : _____
Specimen: _____

INFANT DATA **(12)**
Peds present
□ No   □ Yes
□ Yes, called after delivery
code _____

Apgar scores

	HR	RR	R	T	C	TOT
1 min						
5 min						
10 min						

MECONIUM
□ None   □ Thin/stained
□ Thick   □ Terminal only
□ Wall NP suction on perineum
Intubation for Mec □ No □ Yes
Mec Below Cord □ No □ Yes

RESUSCITATION
□ None/stimulation
□ Mask ventilation
□ Intubation for ventilation
□ Major resuscitation
   (i.e., Umb Cath)
□ Narcotic antagonist given
   ___ mg
□ Surfactant given

_____
Pediatric M.D. signature

New Born ID#:
_____

□ Gross congenital defects

Anomaly: _____

SEX   □ male   □ female
           □ ambiguous

Birth Order ___
   of 1 2 3 4 5

Weight _____ gm

SCN □ NO □ YES

UMBILICAL CORD GASES **(13)**
	pH	BE	pCO2
A	___	___	___
V	___	___	___

DECEASED **(14)**
□ Antepartum
□ Intrapartum ___/___/___ ___:___
□ In LDR/OR ___/___/___ ___:___
□ To path
req # _____
□ To morgue

(15)
RN _____

OB attending _____

OB fellow _____

OB resident 1 _____

OB resident 2 _____

Anesthesia att. _____

Other _____

scrub ORT RN

_____

tient currently undergoing a vaginal trial of labor. *Lacerations* = notes the degree of severity. *Cathed In DR* = catheter in delivery room.

8. Most Recent HCT = hematocrit value

9. Antibiotics Pre Cord Clamp = notes whether antibiotics were given prior to clamping the umbilical cord.

10. Cesarean Delivery Data   *Planned VTOL* = planned vaginal trial of labor. *C/S* = cesarean section. *CPD/FTP* = cephalopelvic disproportion/failure to progress. *Other malpres* = other malpresentation. *FHR* = fetal heart rate. *Foley output* = amount of urine put out during procedure.

11. Other Delivery Information   *Placenta* = notes how the placenta was removed. *Nuchal cord* = part of the umbilical cord is wrapped around the baby's neck. *Cord knot* = a knot in the cord. *EBL* = Estimated blood loss, in cubic centimeters (cc). *Transfusion in DR* = transfusion in delivery room. *Yes, RBC* = packed red blood cells. *Yes, other* = platelets or any other blood products.

12. Infant Data   *Peds present* = notes whether pediatricians were present at the delivery. *Code* = each hospital assigns a color code to identify the   level of pediatric assistance needed. *Apgar scores: HR* = heart rate, *RR* = respiration rate, *R* = reflex response, *T* = muscle tone, *C* = color, *TOT* = total. *Meconium, terminal only* = passing of meconium during delivery. *Wall NP suction on perineum* = plastic tubing attached to a suction outlet in the wall is inserted in baby's nose, mouth, and throat to remove meconium immediately after head is delivered. *Major resuscitation (i.e., Umb Cath)* = catheterization of umbilical artery or vein. *Narcotic antagonist given* = notes whether the baby was given an injection to counteract the effects of a narcotic given to the mother. *Surfactant given* = notes whether a surfactant was needed to prevent lungs from collapsing. *SCN* = Notes if the baby was taken to the special care nursery.

13. Umbilical Cord Gases   These are measurements of the oxygenation of the baby's blood at birth.

14. Deceased   This section is for the rare event of fetal death. *Antepartum* = before labor. *Intrapartum* = during labor. *In LDR/OR* = in labor delivery room or operating room. *To path* = to pathology for autopsy.

15. Attending nurses and physicians   sign or initial here.

. . . . . .

Glossary

Breech presentation—Instead of being in a head-down position, the fetus sits in the pelvis, with buttocks or feet down.

Cephalopelvic disproportion—Literally, "head to pelvis" disproportion, meaning that the fetal head will not fit through the mother's pelvis, either because the head is too big or the pelvis is too small.

Cervical effacement—The cervix, 2–4 centimeters in length, is the cylindrically-shaped bottom of the uterus. When effacement occurs, the length of the cervix decreases, and the tissue is horizontally stretched or "thinned out." If a 3-centimeter-long cervix is 50 percent effaced it means its length has been reduced to 1.5 centimeters.

Classical uterine incision—A vertical incision extending from the top to the bottom of the uterus. This incision, no longer used routinely, confers a much greater risk of uterine rupture in a subsequent labor than a low transverse incision.

Decelerations—Drops in the fetal heart rate that occur during labor.

Doula—A trained female labor companion. Also called a monitrice.

Dystocia—A catchall term meaning abnormal progress of labor and historically listed as a reason for many cesarean sections. The term is falling out of favor because of its vagueness.

Effacement—See cervical effacement.

Endometritis—Inflammation of the uterine lining (the endometrium) due to an intrauterine infection.

External cephalic version—A medical procedure in which an attempt is made to manually turn a fetus from a breech position to a vertex position. It is usually performed after the 37th week of pregnancy.

Fetal bradycardia—A prolonged drop in the fetal heart rate below the normal baseline rate of 100 to 120 beats per minute.

Fetal macrosomia—Large-bodied baby. Though there is no uniform definition, babies weighing more than 4000 grams (8 lbs. 13 oz.) are considered macrosomic by some definitions, while babies weighing 4500 grams (9 lbs. 15 oz.) or more are always considered macrosomic.

Fetal tachycardia—An excessively rapid fetal heart rate, which means the fetal heart has to work harder to extract oxygen from the blood.

Fetopelvic disproportion—See cephalopelvic disproportion.

Fetoscope—A fetal stethoscope; an instrument placed on the mother's abdomen and used to determine the fetal heart rate.

Footling breech presentation—A fetal presentation in which one or both feet of the fetus present first (followed by the buttocks).

Frank breech presentation—A fetal presentation in which the buttocks present first, with the feet extending upwards.

Gravida—A pregnant woman.

Hydramnios—A condition in which there is too much amniotic fluid.

Iatrogenic—A condition induced by a doctor or other medical personnel; often used with regard to "iatrogenic prematurity," meaning prematurity resulting from a cesarean performed before the baby's lungs are mature.

Informed consent—The concept that you have the right to have your questions about the risks and benefits of a procedure and its alternatives answered, and that you have the right to say yes or no to the procedure.

Intermittent auscultation—Intermittent use of the fetoscope during labor to monitor the baby's heart rate.

Intrapartum—During labor or delivery.

Late deceleration—A subtle decline in fetal heart rate after the peak of a contraction; the decline is slow in onset and slow to recover.

Low transverse uterine incision—A low horizontal incision on the uterus; it is preferred in most cesarean deliveries today and confers a lower risk of rupture in a subsequent labor than the classical incision. Note that the skin incision may differ from the uterine incision.

Meconium—Literally, the first fetal bowel movement, which is greenish-brown in color. It can be problematical if the fetus defecates in the amniotic fluid during labor and then inhales fluid containing thick meconium. The passing of meconium in utero may indicate fetal distress.

Multiparous—A woman who has had more than one child.

Myoma—A benign tumor of the uterine muscle tissue, also known as a fibroid tumor.

Myomectomy—The surgical removal of one or more myomas.

Nonreassuring fetal heart rate patterns—A clinical assessment of concern about the baby's condition, based on electronic fetal monitoring.

Nullipara—A woman who has had no children.

Occiputanterior—A fetal position in which the back of the baby's head is against the front of the mother's pelvis. The occipital bone forms the back of the baby's skull, and anterior refers to the front side of the mother. This is a favorable position for successful vaginal delivery.

Occiputposterior—A fetal position in which the back of the baby's head is against the back of the mother's pelvis. The occipital bone forms the back of the baby's skull, and posterior refers to the back side of the mother. This position causes back labor and may make vaginal delivery difficult.

Oligohydramnios—A condition in which there is not enough amniotic fluid.

Perineum—The region from the bottom of the vagina to the anus.

Pitocin— A synthetic form of the naturally occurring hormone oxytocin, which causes contractions. Pitocin is used to induce labor and/or to augment labor when contractions are not sufficient to dilate the cervix.

Placenta—The structure that serves as both lifeline and barrier between mother and fetus. The placenta carries vital nutrients to the fetus from the mother's blood and transports fetal wastes back to the mother's bloodstream for elimination. It also blocks some harmful substances and microorganisms from crossing into the baby's bloodstream.

Placenta accreta—A rare condition in which the placenta implants too firmly in the uterine wall and does not separate spontaneously after the baby is delivered. It can lead to infection and hemorrhage.

Placental abruption—A condition in which the placenta separates partially or completely from the uterine wall during late pregnancy or labor, often requiring cesarean delivery.

Placenta previa—A condition in which the placenta forms across the cervical opening, usually necessitating cesarean delivery.

Preeclampsia—A serious maternal condition, specific to pregnancy and of unknown cause; its symptoms include high blood pressure, excessive and sudden weight gain caused by fluid retention, and protein in the urine.

Primigravida—A woman who is pregnant for the first time.

Prostaglandin gel—A gel used to help induce labor; it has the effect of softening an unripe cervix to make it more favorable for vaginal delivery.

Rectovaginal fistula—A fistula is any abnormal passage between two body parts; a rectovaginal fistula is a narrow opening between the vagina and the rectum that can occur as a result of lacerations incurred by vaginal delivery.

Transverse lie—A fetal position in which the fetus lies across the mother's pelvis.

Umbilical cord prolapse—The descent of the umbilical cord into the birth canal before the baby's presenting part, which can compress the cord and compromise the baby's oxygen supply. It is more common in breech or transverse presentation and requires cesarean delivery.

Vertex presentation—A fetal position in which the fetus is head down.

Index

Hunter House
Women's Health

ONCE A MONTH: The *Original* Premenstrual Syndrome Handbook — 5th revised edition *by* Katharina Dalton, M.D.
Premenstrual syndrome may be the world's most common condition—surveys have shown that as many as 75% of women complain of at least one medical symptom of premenstrual syndrome. Dr. Katharina Dalton pioneered the diagnosis and treatment of PMS. In ONCE A MONTH she describes premenstrual symptoms, the hormonal changes that cause them, and the best medical and self-help treatments for dealing with them. The new fifth edition contains a chapter on PMS and pregnancy, added informaion about the role of diet in managing PMS symptoms, and personal stories of women who have lived with PMS for several years.

"Dalton is amply qualified to make the diagnosis."
—NEWSWEEK

288 pages ... 37 illus ... Paperback $11.95 ... Hardcover $21.95

FROM ACUPRESSURE TO ZEN: An Encyclopedia of Natural Therapies *by* Barbara Nash
Natural therapies make a wonderful complement to traditional medicine. This book provides clear descriptions of over 70 therapies, from ayurvedic medicine and Bach flower remedies to homeopathy, T'ai Chi, and Zen. Each entry includes information on the therapy's origin, how it helps, and how traditional doctors feel about it. It also lists more than 150 ailments and suggests natural therapies to treat them. Special sections cover pregnancy, family health, and sexual problems.

336 pages ... 24 illus. ... Paperback $15.95 ... Hard cover $25.95

THE NEW A-TO-Z OF WOMEN'S HEALTH
by Christine Ammer
An up-to-date work with over 1000 detailed, expert entries covering all aspects of a woman's health. A cross-reference system and subject guide make it easy for women and professionals to consult, and the broad list of topics includes: pregnancy, childbirth, and birth control • drugs, medication, fitness, and vitamins • cholesterol and diet • chronic disease and disabilities • sexuality and sexually transmitted diseases.

"The coverage is more extensive than that of *The New Our Bodies, Ourselves* and more current than that of Felicia Stewart's *Understanding Your Body*." — BOOKLIST

496 pages ... 10 illus ... Paperback $16.95

Prices subject to change . . . to order please see last page

ORDER FORM

10% DISCOUNT on orders of $20 or more —
20% DISCOUNT on orders of $50 or more —
30% DISCOUNT on orders of $250 or more —
On cost of books for fully prepaid orders

NAME

ADDRESS

CITY/STATE   ZIP/POSTCODE

PHONE   COUNTRY (outside U.S.)

TITLE	QTY		PRICE	TOTAL
Vaginal Birth after Cesarean	I	@	$ 12.95	
A-to-Z of Pregnancy and Childbirth	I	@	$ 16.95	
Fertility Awarenes Handbook	I	@	$ 11.95	
Getting Pregnant and Staying Pregnant	I	@	$ 14.95	
List other titles below:				
	I	@	$	
	I	@	$	
	I	@	$	
	I	@	$	
	I	@	$	
	I	@	$	
	I	@	$	

Shipping costs:
*First book: $2.50
($6.00 outside U.S.)*
*Each additional book:
$1.00 ($2.00 outside
U.S.)*
*For UPS rates and
bulk orders call us at
(510) 865-5282*

SUBTOTAL	
Less discount @_____%	( )
TOTAL COST OF BOOKS	
Calif. residents add sales tax	
Shipping & handling	
TOTAL ENCLOSED	
Please pay in U.S. funds only	

☐ Check   ☐ Money Order   ☐ Visa   ☐ M/C   ☐ Discover

Card # _____ Exp date _____

Signature _____

Complete and mail to:

Hunter House Inc., Publishers
P.O. Box 2914, Alameda CA 94501-0914
Orders: 1-800-266-5592
Phone (510) 865-5282 Fax (510) 865-4295 E-mail: ordering@hunterhouse.com

☐ Check here to receive our FREE book catalog

VBA 5/96